T0244258

"Pascal Baudar has long served as an inspiration to me as both a forager and a fermenter. With *Wildcrafted Vinegars*, he once again delivers on the promise of bringing the outdoors inside. On its surface, this book is a fantastic guide to crafting a whole pantry's worth of staple vinegars and condiments to ameliorate your cooking, but at its core, it's a practical call to action through recipes that turn you into an agent of ecological remediation, wherever you might live. A must-have for any avid fermenter!"

—David Zilber, chef and food scientist; coauthor of
the *New York Times* bestseller *The Noma Guide to Fermentation*

"From apple scraps to mugwort to bountiful berries, Baudar brings vinegar-making past the boundaries of our ordinary home pantries and out into the great wide open. Anything is a possible flavoring here, be it roots, herbs, or stems. As with his other books, Baudar once again enlightens us to the fact that flavor is found from the forest floor to the tips of the trees, and even takes inspiration from humdrum supermarket shelves to make vinegars that shine."

—Michael Harlan Turkell, award-winning food photographer,
author of *Acid Trip: Travels in the World of Vinegar*

"Pascal Baudar continues to lead his readers down a path that connects them to their landscapes, whether urban or wild, through culinary exploration—this time through the power of sour. *Wildcrafted Vinegars* is a visually striking invitation to explore flavorful condiments, preserves, and quick pickles from unexpected and often overlooked seeds and 'weeds.'"

—Kirsten K. Shockey, author of *Homebrewed Vinegar*,
Fermented Vegetables, and other fermentation titles

"*Wildcrafted Vinegars* is another outstanding fermentation guide from Pascal Baudar. With wonderful clarity and a variety of flexible approaches, Pascal simultaneously demystifies the vinegar-making process and inspires the imagination with its infinite possibilities."

—Sandor Ellix Katz, fermentation revivalist,
author of *The Art of Fermentation*

"Baudar's approaches to vinegar making are serious and whimsical at the same time. A true pioneer in the world of fermentation, he is pushing the boundaries on our future food production, while illuminating the past and the very origins of one of the most important products in human history. The wealth of ideas and information contained in *Wildcrafted Vinegars* cannot be overstated, and this book has a place in every kitchen."

—Harry Rosenblum, author of *Vinegar Revival*

"Pascal Baudar has once again tapped into the spirit of the forest and open spaces in this paean to all things pungent. A love letter to *Acetobacter* in the wild, it will have you thinking about vinegar in a whole new light—not only as essential in the kitchen but really quite easy to make yourself, too."

—Ken Albala, professor of history, University of the Pacific

"Having closely followed the musings and teachings of Mr. Baudar through his previous works, I have found that his creations emanate from an uncommon combination of scientific experimentation and culinary curiosity, always showing great reverence for traditional foodways.

"In this fun book, Baudar, with his playful spirit of adventure, brings us on yet another creative quest that appeals to both the chef and forager in all of us.

"While drawing us into the rarified ancient world of fermentations and *Acetobacter* (the 'mothers' of vinegar), Baudar also keeps one foot firmly planted in the reality of our modern world's fragile ecology. A few pages of this book could serve as the most practical guide to vinegar production (including the use of fruit flies to initiate a wild fermentation!), but the remaining pages serve as an invaluable compendium of wild food flavors and recipes.

"This book will be a fixture on my kitchen bookshelf where rainy-day culinary projects begin."

—Evan Mallett, chef/owner, Black Trumpet Bistro;
author of *Black Trumpet*

"Pascal Baudar, long-time wild food forager extraordinaire and vinegar savant, has created a book that will revolutionize the vinegar world. *Wildcrafted Vinegars* is an acetic A–Z of fermentation advice and lore, beautifully illustrated with his helpful photographs, to guide you to new levels of culinary experimentation. As a fellow vinegar maker and lover, it left me totally in awe of his expertise and passion . . ."

—Andy Harris, CVO (chief vinegar officer), Vinegar Shed

Wildcrafted Vinegars

Also by Pascal Baudar

The New Wildcrafted Cuisine:
Exploring the Exotic Gastronomy of Local Terroir

The Wildcrafting Brewer:
Creating Unique Drinks and Boozy Concoctions
from Nature's Ingredients

Wildcrafted Fermentation:
Exploring, Transforming, and Preserving
the Wild Flavors of Your Local Terroir

Wildcrafted Vinegars

Making and Using Unique Acetic Acid Ferments
for Quick Pickles, Hot Sauces, Soups,
Salad Dressings, Pastes, Mustards, and More

PASCAL BAUDAR

Chelsea Green Publishing
White River Junction, Vermont
London, UK

Project Manager: Alexander Bullett
Developmental Editor: Natalie Wallace
Copy Editor: Diane Durrett
Proofreader: Angela Boyle
Indexer: Joel Kaemmerlen
Designer: Melissa Jacobson

Printed in the United States of America.
First printing October 2022.
10 9 8 7 6 5 4 3 2 1   22 23 24 25 26

Our Commitment to Green Publishing
Chelsea Green sees publishing as a tool for cultural change and ecological stewardship. We strive to align our book manufacturing practices with our editorial mission and to reduce the impact of our business enterprise in the environment. We print our books and catalogs on chlorine-free recycled paper, using vegetable-based inks whenever possible. This book may cost slightly more because it was printed on paper that contains recycled fiber, and we hope you'll agree that it's worth it. *Wildcrafted Vinegars* was printed on paper supplied by Versa Press that is made of recycled materials and other controlled sources.

ISBN 978-1-64502-114-8 (paperback) | ISBN 978-1-64502-115-5 (ebook)

Library of Congress Cataloging-in-Publication Data is available upon request.

Chelsea Green Publishing
85 North Main Street, Suite 120
White River Junction, Vermont USA

Somerset House
London, UK

www.chelseagreen.com

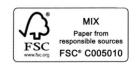

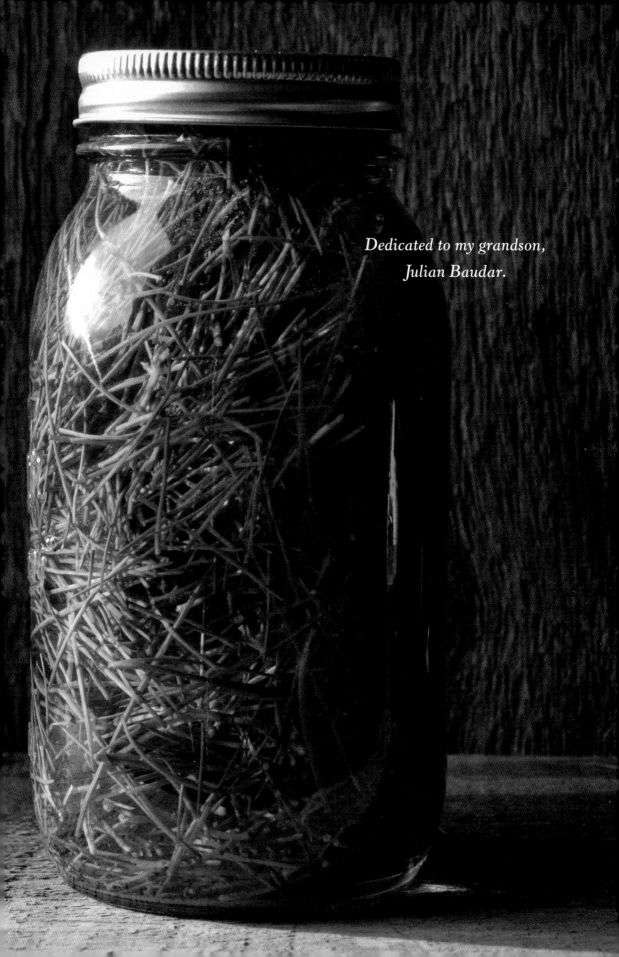

Dedicated to my grandson,
Julian Baudar.

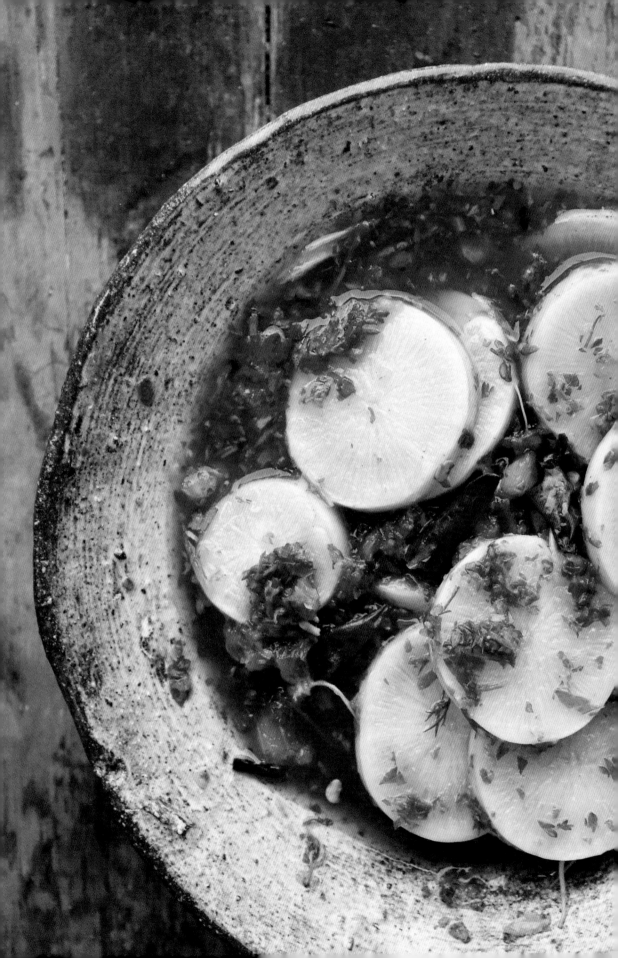

CONTENTS

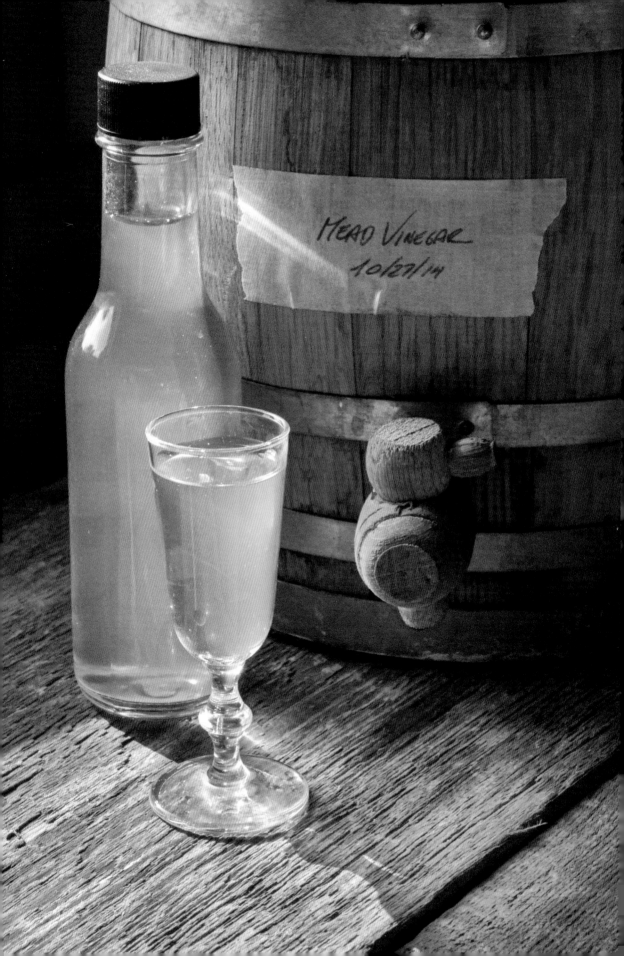

Why Vinegars?

After I finished writing my last book, *Wildcrafted Fermentation*, I had another book idea in mind. I had just purchased an RV with the intention of expanding my horizons by traveling across North America and connecting with like-minded people.

The concept for that next book was to look at environmental issues and explore the possibility of a wildcrafted cuisine that would be beneficial, not just sustainable, for the environment. Sounds incredible, but it's actually quite possible.

In Los Angeles, where I lived at the time, I was surrounded by a huge quantity of wild edibles that are considered invasive or non-native, so much so that our local hills turn completely yellow around April due to the large amount of flowering Mediterranean mustard (*Hirschfeldia incana*) and black mustard (*Brassica nigra*).

The number of wild edibles was quite mind-boggling! We're talking about more than 8 varieties of wild mustards, dandelion (*Taraxacum officinale*), common stinging nettle (*Urtica dioica*), chickweed (*Stellaria media*), wild radish (*Raphanus raphanistrum*), curly dock (*Rumex crispus*), watercress (*Nasturtium officinale*), wild chervil (*Anthriscus sylvestris*), and countless others.

Quite a few of these plants are cultivated in some countries, but locally they are simply viewed as unwanted and non-native, and sometimes labeled invasive. There are no positive solutions to deal with the "problem"—it's either chemicals and herbicides or what is called "habitat restoration," whereby plants are uprooted and then thrown away.

I know it's not even a blip on the radar of environmentalists or city administrators, but from my perspective, one of the biggest food wastes in the Los Angeles area is the nonuse of those edible, unwanted plants that cover the local hills and vast fields surrounding the city. This waste is sad to contemplate given that we also have a large number of people who cannot afford nutritious and organic food.

So, from my perspective, the concept for this new book was to look for positive solutions to environmental challenges rather than negative ones. How can we create a nourishing cuisine that has a positive impact on both the environment and our own health? I think it's a dialogue worth having. I always say that my job is to plant seeds in people's heads.

But why am I talking about all of this in a book about vinegar?

Most people don't realize it, but if you intend to make wild food a substantial part of your diet or want to create interesting dishes all year long, then wildcrafting is all about food preservation. The use of natural methods to preserve wild edibles and rediscover long-lost flavors is crucial, and, as foragers, we are the keepers of culinary traditions that are slowly disappearing. One such method—fermentation—has been a centerpiece of my previous books. *The Wildcrafting Brewer* is about alcoholic fermentation, which involves the breakdown of sugars by yeasts. In *Wildcrafted Fermentation*, the focus shifts to lacto-fermentation, or the breakdown of sugars by bacteria that produce lactic acid. Vinegar is created by a third form of fermentation, acetic fermentation, which occurs when *Acetobacter* bacteria convert alcohols into acetic acid, or vinegar.

I realized I just could not avoid writing this book—about the missing fermentation form—before going on to the next. Vinegar is essential to wildcrafting, and *Acetobacter*, such as lactobacteria or wild yeast, can be found in your environment. If you know how to make your own vinegars, you can do much more than just preserve the harvest; you can also create an incredible array of tasty side dishes, condiments, and even drinks featuring truly local flavors.

Preserving the Harvest, Preserving Knowledge

With the convenience of supermarkets and easy access to farmed ingredients, it's easy to forget that food preservation is at the heart of much of the food we eat. Look at the grocery bags of the average consumer—the vast majority of the contents are preserved goods such as sodas, pasta, beer, wine, chips, cold-stored fish or meat, frozen food, cheeses, canned soups, condiments like hot sauce or mustard, and so on.

It's no different with wild food; thus, the basics of food preservation and how to apply it to wild edibles should be high on the list of "know-how" for any forager.

The sad part is, basic food preservation techniques are not taught anymore and the knowledge is lost for the average person. I remember giving a class to around 30 students at Santa Monica College a couple of years ago.

I asked if anyone in the class knew about food preservation techniques. One student, of Korean descent, told me that she knew how to make kimchi. No one else had a clue.

I found it fascinating that here we had 30 students highly educated in all kinds of complicated subjects, but, aside from one person, no one knew the basics of preserving food.

If you think about it, it is completely backward. A few generations ago our ancestors knew how to preserve the harvest in all kinds of creative ways, but in the present time we rely on a food system all set up for us. Should the food system collapse, even the brightest minds would not know what to do.

To make it worse, look at all the unhealthy and processed food on the store shelves: overly sweet sodas, meat from animals raised in dubious conditions, vegetables sprayed with pesticides unless you pay a premium for organic ones, and excessive salt and various additives in preserved hams and cheeses. The last time I shopped, I checked the label of a cheese I purchased; I had no idea what 80 percent of the ingredients were. Wasn't cheese once made of milk, cheese cultures, enzymes, and salt?

Unless you buy local food from sources you know, you are dealing with a capitalistic system based on mass consumption. Factors such as speed and profit are considered more important than consumers' health.

I understand that a "system" had to be set in place to feed a growing population and ensure food safety. But, when looking at the CDC site in February 2022, they estimated that every year 1 in 6 Americans (or 48 million people) get sick from foodborne diseases, 128,000 are hospitalized, and 3,000 die.* You decide if you would call that a success.

It is becoming increasingly necessary to rely on our own knowledge for health and safety, as without it, we are slaves to a system. Our grocery stores may appear to offer the "freedom of choice," but the system decides what is available for purchase and at what price. That's why you can find only 5 types of potatoes in the store while over 4,000 varieties exist in the world. As for vinegars, you're pretty much stuck with 5 or 6 types, including the cheap balsamic imitation made with regular vinegar, sweetener, and colorants. Good luck trying to find blackberry or elderberry wine vinegar on a shelf.

But let's forget the doomsday scenario. For a wildcrafter, traditional food preservation expands the possibilities for the creation of healthy and flavorful dishes. It also allows you yearlong enjoyment of the harvest collected during times of plenty, which is usually only a few months of the year.

---

* Centers for Disease Control and Prevention, "Fast Facts about Food Poisoning," last updated May 11, 2021, cdc.gov/foodsafety/food-poisoning.html.

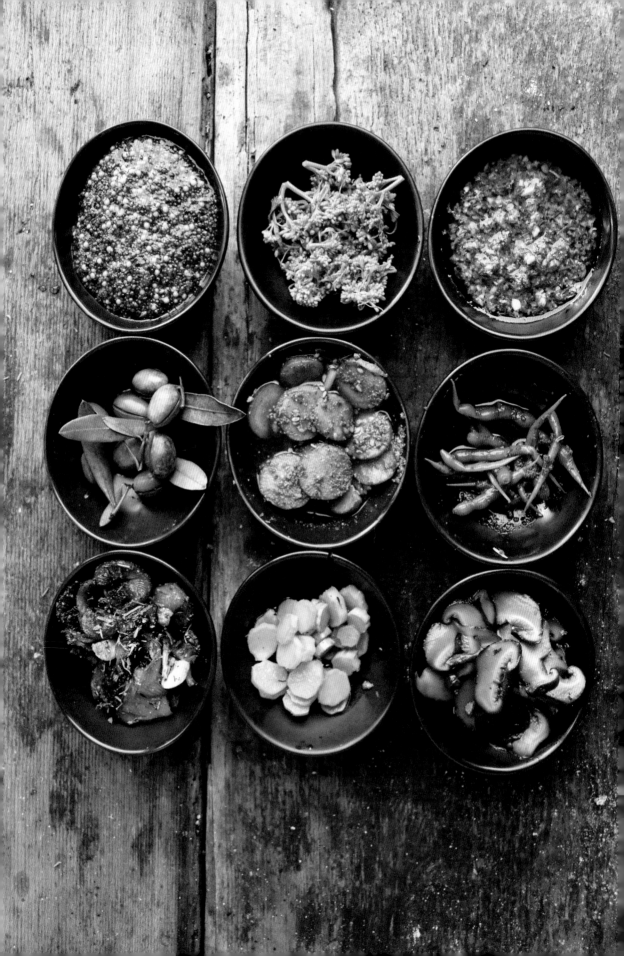

In Los Angeles, the local wilderness turns into a desert during the summer; thus, my main harvest time is from December to June. Meanwhile, most northern states have little to forage but snow during the winter.

Foraging is not like going to the supermarket, where you'll find tomatoes and other vegetables all year long. Food in nature will be available only for a couple of months (or less) and often goes through different phases, during which different parts of the plant become available as food. I'll forage delicious black mustard sprouts in late winter or early spring. Then, as time passes, I'll collect the black mustard leaves, stems, roots, flowers, and finally seeds. Each ingredient can be preserved in a different way. For example, the leaves and roots can be fermented, stems pickled in vinegar, and seeds dehydrated to make a sort of Dijon mustard condiment later. Such a process is true of most wild food.

Food preservation allows you to create extraordinary flavors and preserves that can become gourmet food in their own right. In some cultures, side dishes are often the most important element of daily food consumption (*banchan* in Korea, for example, or *tsukemono* in Japan).

In Belgium, where I grew up, gourmet preserves showed up as appetizers or finger foods during special celebrations such as weddings and holidays. Most of these preserves—smoked salmon, scrumptious pâtés, pickled onions and cornichons (mini gherkin cucumbers), caviar, and so on—are rooted in traditional food preservation techniques.

Countless cultures recognize the importance of savory preserves, and a feast is often defined by the multitude of side dishes. Spain is the land of tapas; and in China and Lebanon, meals usually consist of one main dish and many other small dishes laid out across the table.

Unlike store-bought foodstuff, true traditional preserves are often alive, and therefore a good source of probiotics. We're talking fermented vegetables, pickles made from raw homemade vinegars, olives cured without the need for lye, artisan cheeses made with natural cultures, homemade beers and wines brewed with wild yeast, and much more!

If you want to explore a cuisine based on your environment and share it with others, the ability to create your own vinegars using local ingredients is vital.

When I was giving my plant walks before the 2020 pandemic, we would always enjoy a large feast at the end of each class featuring the plants we saw during the walk. Probably an average of 10 to 15 flavorful dishes and drinks were available for each participant to taste and enjoy. For most of the

Wildcrafted vinegar-based pickles.

dishes, I combined traditional food preservation techniques with fresh wild ingredients.

Without homemade vinegars, I would have never been able to investigate my local flavors so deeply to create condiments and dishes that could not be purchased at the supermarket—wild mustard seeds pickled in white elderberry wine vinegar, feral olives cured with prickly pear vinegar, oyster mushrooms (*Pleurotus ostreatus*) preserved in a beer vinegar made with traditional bitter herbs collected from the same forest, and so many others!

I hope this book will provide you with ideas and inspiration to explore the infinite culinary possibilities of your own unique environment.

How to Use This Book

This book is about creating homemade vinegars using wildcrafted or store-bought ingredients. You will also find recipes for flavoring vinegars; creating drinks, sauces, and quick pickles; and more.

I use very traditional and simple methods to create my vinegars—the equipment necessary to make them is commonly available. You probably have them in your kitchen already. So there's no need to order special tools. This is pretty much the way vinegars have been made for centuries. There are other ways to make vinegars using a more modern approach and tools that can speed up the process, but I choose to let the flavors develop just like nature intended.

A lot of the plants, fruits, and berries used in the recipes in this book, with a few exceptions, can be found all over North America and Europe. A lot of them are also considered non-native and often invasive. It is totally possible to create a cuisine based on traditional preservation techniques that is beneficial for the environment, and vinegar making can be an integral part of the process.

As with all of my books, think of the recipes as ideas and concepts that you can apply to your own local flora.

Have fun and create!

On Picking Wild Plants, or Foraging

Like many of our human activities, foraging can be done for good or evil; it can help the environment or intensify sustainability issues. Over the years I've learned to streamline my activities so as to minimize my impact on nature. It's been a learning curve with trials and errors, but these days I actually think foraging can be done in such a way that allows you to help your local environment. This is accomplished by removing non-native plants (pretty much 90 percent of what I pick) and by sustainably harvesting or growing the native plants you need. As far as I can remember, I pretty much replanted all the native plants I used for recipes in this book, in much larger quantities than I'll ever use, mostly on private lands owned by friends.

You don't need to be a fanatic tree hugger to see that our planet faces real problems such as pollution, climate change (natural or not), human expansion, loss of natural habitat, species extinction, and the like. We absolutely need to be part of the solution, and this responsibility even applies to the simple act of picking wild plants. We must make sure that our picking wild plants for food, drinks, or medicine is done carefully, with environmental health and integrity in mind.

Picking plants and berries for food or making drinks can connect us back to nature: It is a sacred link that, as a species, we all share. We are here because our ancestors had a very intimate relationship with nature, knew which plants to use for food or medicine, and in many instances knew how to sustainably interact with their wild environment. No matter where we live, whether we recognize it or not, it's part of our cultural DNA.

I personally don't think the impulse to protect nature at all costs with a look-don't-touch mentality will work. Growing up in Belgium, I came by my love for nature through a deep interaction with my wild surroundings. If you truly love something, you will take care of it and make sure it is still there for generations to come.

When I was a kid, raising animals, growing food in our garden, and picking wild berries, nuts, and plants weren't considered weird or special activities; they were a normal part of life. Elders would pass their knowledge on to the next generation. In many modernized countries, this cycle of transferring knowledge has been lost. Very valuable and nutritious foods such as dandelion, mallow, and other plants are looked upon as "weeds," and TV commercials gladly promote the use of toxic chemicals to destroy them. The people I've seen trashing the wilderness are the product of our current society. If you don't know or understand the value of something, you simply won't care for it.

So do it the right way! Respect the environment, learn which plants are rare or illegal to pick, don't forage plants in protected areas (natural preserves and the like), work with native plant nurseries, and educate yourself on how to grow native plants and remove non-natives.

If you take from nature, work with her and make sure you always plant more than you'll ever take. That way future generations will have the same creative opportunities you presently have—or more.

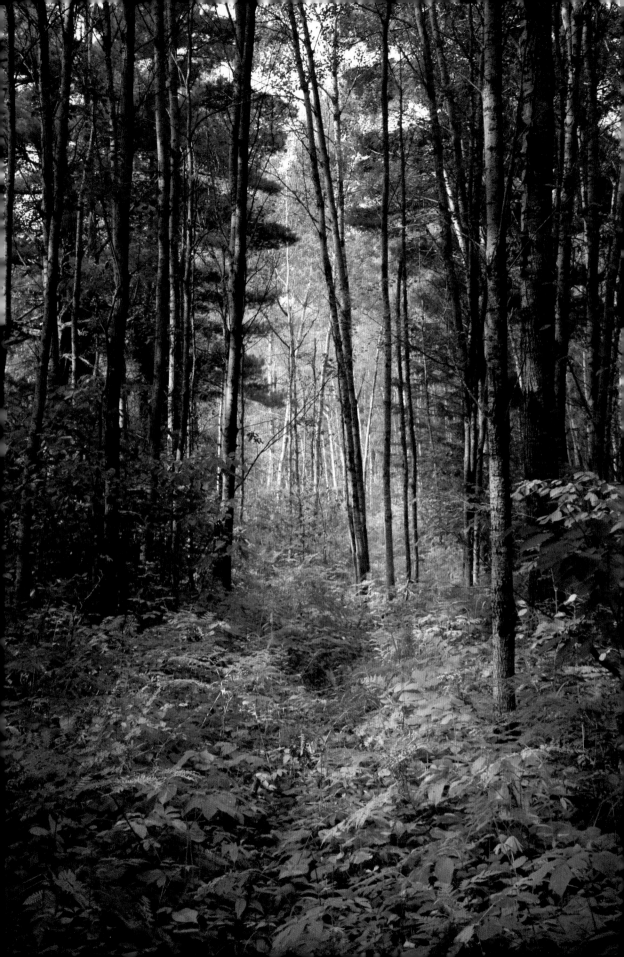

CHAPTER 1

Vinegar Basics: Making Vinegars at Home

W e'll probably never find out exactly when vinegar was "discovered." While its true origins will likely remain lost in prehistory, I think vinegar probably appeared in various parts of the world independently based on the research I did on ancestral alcoholic beverages for *The Wildcrafting Brewer*.

The histories of alcohol and vinegar are tightly bound together. In my fertile imagination, I can see how some of those old prehistoric shamanic brews fermented with wild yeast, local honey, berries, and plants would have eventually turned into vinegar as part of a natural process. The bacteria responsible for turning alcohol to vinegar (*Acetobacter*) are usually part of the same microbiome as the wild yeasts that convert sugars to alcohol. Once the wild yeasts do their work, the *Acetobacter* take over and perform the second conversion.

Nevertheless, the first known mention of vinegar making and its uses appears in ancient Babylonian scrolls from around 5000 BC, which is quite early in recorded history. At that time, vinegar was made from beverages such as fig or date wines and all-grain beers. The next discovery of vinegar in the historical record came when traces of vinegar were found in 3,000-year-old Egyptian urns.

From that point on, which we know thanks to the evidence found in written documents, vinegar was quite popular. It was most commonly consumed as a beverage, but it was also used as a food preservative and for its medicinal properties. One of the main drinks in ancient Greece, called *oxycrate*, was made by combining vinegar with water and honey. It's very similar to what we call a *shrub* in modern times. The Romans had their own vinegar-based drink, called *posca*, which was composed of red wine vinegar, water, spices, and honey.

But the golden age of vinegar came in the late Middle Ages with the worldwide advent of an active maritime and land-based commercial trade.

Vinegar developed into an important commodity, used to preserve food-stuff, create drinks, make condiments and sauces, and more. The French town of Orléans became known as an important production center, and their vinegar-making method was a standard for several centuries.

The fermentation process behind the production of vinegar was never truly understood until 1864, when Louis Pasteur discovered that *Acetobacter* bacteria were responsible for the conversion of alcohol to acetic acid.

Armed with that knowledge, nineteenth- and particularly twentieth-century experimenters developed new methods to accelerate the fermentation process. This was accomplished primarily by increasing the amount of oxygen and the speed at which it was supplied to the bacteria.

Today, instead of taking weeks to produce, vinegar can be made within a couple of days thanks to technology. Those are the vinegars you will find in the supermarket.

But, interestingly enough, many high-quality vinegars are still made in the good old ways—by allowing time for the natural fermentation process to slowly transform the alcoholic beverage into a savory acidic liquid, which is sometimes aged in wooden barrels for years before consumption. This book is based on that philosophy of letting Mother Nature do her magical work and, in the end, enjoying her delicious creation.

Wildcrafted Vinegars

When I was working on *The Wildcrafting Brewer*, which is about brewing and fermenting with wild yeast, one of my biggest discoveries was this: In our modern world, we really like to complicate things.

If you think about it, beer originated from the simple concept of boiling bitter herbs (mugwort [*Artemisia douglasiana*], yarrow [*Achillea millefolium*], hops, and so forth) with a source of sugar (malted grains). The mixture was then cooled down and fermented with the available wild yeast found in nature, then enjoyed.

Looking back in time, many of those old fermented beverages didn't fit specific categories or labels such as beer, wine, mead, and so on. People created boozy, tasty drinks with whatever their environment provided, mixing various sources of sugar if necessary. But nowadays, most of our alcoholic beverages are neatly categorized.

The advantage of categories is that you can create and enforce rules on how beverages of a certain category *must* be produced, require that ingredients be purchased from specific sources (the church or state in the old days), put together precise "scientific methods" and a whole education system required to learn them, sell expensive equipment, and tax the final product, too. Lots of money is involved when things are made more complex.

Humans are very good at "improving" nature; we like to be in charge and control things. And when we're done perfecting the process to our liking, we look back at how things were done in the past and call it primitive, imperfect, archaic, insisting that what we do now is so much better because we control every part of the process.

During my research I read a book about commercial vinegar production, and right there in the beginning the authors mentioned the "inferior product" of homemade vinegars created using simple methods. It wasn't a bad book—there was a lot of interesting and solid information in it—but the manufacturing process described was very controlled and scientific. It required all sorts of equipment to achieve modern "perfection" and, per the authors, "superior flavors."

I know, I know . . . I'm ranting a little bit. Maybe I'm getting cranky as I get older.

If you think about it, it's all just perspective. There is really nothing wrong with taking a modern approach to producing something. In the commercial setting it's often necessary to have a tightly controlled production system so you can create a product (beer, wine, vinegar) with a specific, consistent flavor. And for good reasons! You probably would not like taste variations in your favorite beer or wine.

But I think there is a bit of arrogance in the assumption that, without tight supervision and control, we will achieve an inferior product, as though nature isn't capable of producing something decent without our input.

You'll find a similar attitude with cheese production. A lot of the cheeses available on the shelves in North American supermarkets are quite "civilized" compared to homemade or artisanal cheeses. Growing up in Belgium, I remember that some of our artisan cheeses had very complex flavors and pungency. Some of these cheeses could even be described as having barnyard qualities. They're probably illegal to import to the United States!

And so, I'll happily disagree with some vinegar "experts" who think that strict control and modern methods are the way to go. In fact, I view some imperfections as desirable qualities in many of my wilder acidic creations.

I prefer to work with nature instead of controlling it. With wildcrafted vinegars, we go back in time to rediscover the long-lost flavors of simply-made vinegars. Imperfect as they may be from a modern perspective, they are beautiful and delicious in their own right. We become natural alchemists, working with nature instead of trying to control it.

In nature, things are constantly changing. A mugwort beer made in spring will taste different than one beer made in fall. Nature is unpredictable. You can embrace that fact and work with it. It's like dancing with someone—it's about teamwork, knowing when to let go and when to lead. There are elements in natural processes that can't be found in scientific methods, such as understanding how the seasons and the land can affect flavors and gaining personal intuition from having a special connection with the environment.

And finally, the beauty of wildcrafted vinegars is in the infinite array of possible creations, each of which will be unique and a true representation of your terroir. For example, you can turn your elderberry wine into vinegar, then infuse that vinegar with dehydrated elderberries, doubling the flavor. You can't buy something like that at the store.

Join the dark side and begin your adventure with wild, untamed, uncivilized, and superb flavors.

Making Vinegar from Scratch

When I started looking at traditional food preservation techniques, which was before the internet and search engines were popular, making your own vinegar at home was a big mystery. It seemed that you had to have special connections to people who had some sort of bacteria culture they called a mother, and those people were probably part of a shady, cultish fermentation society that kept its location and practice a secret.

This must have been the case, as I could not find anyone around me with information, and so I kept buying vinegar from the grocery store. It wasn't until I started making my own wines and beers that I finally understood that fermentation was a simple, natural process. Well, sort of . . .

I had a friend who gifted me some elderberry wine every year, and it would always turn into vinegar within a couple of weeks. It was a big mystery to me until I found out that she had little to no experience in making alcoholic drinks and would simply pour the juice in a large bottle to ferment, leaving the bottle open and unprotected (no airlock or cork). It's fine to do this if you intend to drink the wine quite young, but not if you intend to age it.

One by-product of her open fermentation was found at the bottom of the bottles. I always discovered a decent number of dead fruit flies there, which was kind of gross, but it also made sense: The flies were attracted by the fermenting wine, and I assume that some of them were victims of accidental drowning after a night of heavy drinking.

Seriously, though, it took me a while to figure it out. But right there were two keys for her successful, albeit unintentional, artisanal vinegar-making operation. The first key was the fact that her elderberry wine fermentation was made from raw juice (European method), meaning there was wild yeast present on the berries. You'll recall that *Acetobacter*, the bacteria responsible for making vinegar, is normally part of the same microbiome as wild yeast.

Due to her lack of experience, she also didn't use enough sugar to end up with a very alcoholic drink, which was perfect for vinegar making.

The second key was revealed to me by accident while I was researching ancestral alcoholic fermentation. I found out that fruit flies (*Drosophila melanogaster*) were also called vinegar flies—not just because they are attracted to vinegar and alcohol but because they often have *Acetobacter* as part of their gut microbiota and on their body. That was my eureka moment. In essence, the accidental addition of fruit flies helped the vinegar-making process along.

Don't laugh! My first vinegar mother (a jellylike substance that forms at the top of the alcoholic beverage) was made by infecting some of my mugwort beer with fruit flies. I kept the method ultra-simple: I left a jar of beer outside, and in the warm Southern California weather, I had a fruit fly pool party going on within 30 minutes. An hour later I placed the lid on top, screwed it on quickly, then shook the jar a bit and ended up with around 20 fruit flies in the brew.

In a few hours, once the flies had sunk to the bottom of the jar, I unscrewed the lid and secured a clean paper towel over the top with a rubber band, as the vinegar-making process needs oxygen. A week later my brew started to smell slightly like vinegar, and within 4 to 5 weeks I had a beautiful vinegar mother on top.

I experimented much more with this method, which I explain later in this chapter (see Method 3: Fruit Fly Vinegar). Gross or not, it works quite well. I didn't want to include that specific vinegar in any culinary creations due to the dead flies inside, but I used the mother vinegar as a culture starter to "infect" some of my other fermented beverages and turn them into vinegar. To this date, I still have some vinegars made with that original mother.

But I'm already going too fast here. Let's slow down and look at the fundamentals first, so we understand what we're dealing with.

What Is Vinegar?

The answer is super simple: It's just water and acetic acid.

It's a natural step in "wild" fermentation. Vinegar is the theoretical end result whether you do a raw fermentation—such as with the example of my elderberry wine, where wild yeast and *Acetobacter* are present on the fruit— or you create a wild yeast starter and use it to ferment your wine, beer, mead, or similar alcoholic beverage (see Making a Wild Yeast Starter).

Does this conversion of alcohol into vinegar occur all the time? It really depends on several main conditions. You need these 3 factors present to make vinegar:

1. The alcoholic liquid should have access to air. *Acetobacter* thrive in oxygen-rich environments, so a closed container such as a corked bottle is not conducive to vinegar production.
2. The temperature in the environment where the vinegar is made should be around 70 to 95°F (21–35°C). The ideal temperature for bacteria growth is between 77 and 85°F (25–30°C). A vinegar fermentation usually takes 3 to 4 weeks at a temperature of around 80°F (26°C).
3. For home production, the alcoholic content of the beverage you're fermenting is best between 5 and 9 percent.

These variables explain why many wild alcoholic ferments don't turn into vinegar over time, which I guess is a good thing if you didn't want to make vinegar in the first place.

With all 3 factors present, you can take several approaches to start making your own vinegar. I always tell my students that their first goal should be to have an active homemade culture; from that foundation, it's much easier to create more vinegar.

An *active culture* is a raw, unpasteurized vinegar with a mother or live vinegar bacteria (*Acetobacter*) in it. A vinegar mother is a by-product of the fermentation process. A mother is composed mostly of cellulose and bacteria, and the presence of this by-product is a good indication that the fermentation process is active. (I write more about this in "The Mother of Vinegar," page 26).

A mother with a bit of the original unpasteurized vinegar can be used as a starter to create more vinegar. From experience, every mother created will be unique. I've had starters that turned an alcoholic beverage into vinegar quite fast, while others were more sluggish despite the same ambient temperature.

I use three main methods to create a batch of homemade vinegar, and thus, my starter for future vinegars:

1. Introduce the culture from a friend or a commercial source.
2. Create a culture as a natural evolution of the fermentation process.
3. Introduce *Acetobacter* into the alcoholic beverage through a natural source.

The first method consists of obtaining raw vinegar, be it from a commercial source or a friend. The commercial versions are usually advertised as "raw vinegar with the mother." Very often you won't see any mother of vinegar in the bottle, but *Acetobacter* are present. Obtaining some raw vinegar with a bit of vinegar mother from a friend falls in the same category. With this living culture, you can use the vinegar as a starter to create more. This method is highly successful *if* the culture is still alive in the vinegar. I had a couple of failed attempts with a specific batch, and I suspect the failure occurred because the culture inside wasn't alive anymore.

The second method is a bit more complex because you must create the alcoholic beverage that you're starting with. This involves making a wild yeast fermentation with a specific amount of alcohol, then letting it turn naturally into vinegar due to the *Acetobacter* already present in the liquid. Failures with this method can occur when the beverage simply doesn't turn into vinegar, which sometimes is a mystery. But most of the time it will work.

The third method is the crazy one: We "infect" the alcoholic beverage with fruit or vinegar flies on purpose, using the *Acetobacter* present on the flies as the starter culture.

No need to be all serious about it—this should be viewed as a fun project. The idea is to successfully create your first culture starter at home using one or all three of these methods. From there, it's much easier to make more, and success is pretty much guaranteed.

Let's get started!

METHOD 1: USING UNPASTEURIZED VINEGAR AS A STARTER

Using unpasteurized vinegar is the easiest method to start making your own vinegar at home. The first essential ingredient is raw vinegar. It doesn't need to be a red wine vinegar—the Bragg brand of unpasteurized apple cider vinegar works well. I haven't really tried other brands, but they should work, too. The unpasteurized vinegar will be your culture starter to create the vinegar.

The second essential ingredient is red wine. For your first attempt I suggest you use store-bought red wine. From there, you can experiment with other alcoholic beverages. No need to purchase an expensive wine—my favorite red wine vinegar is made with the cheapest wine I could find at the supermarket. Don't use white wine or sparkling wine yet—those are a bit more complex. Stick to regular red wine.

Remember that your alcoholic beverage should be between 5 and 9 percent alcohol to start with; thus, you need to look at the label to determine the alcohol percentage of the wine you purchased. For example, the wine I normally use is 12 percent alcohol and the bottle has a volume of 1 quart (1 L). The alcohol content is therefore too high to make vinegar (as will be the case with most every bottle of wine). So you need to dilute it. I usually add 16 ounces (0.5 L) of water and end up with 8 percent alcohol.

The math is simple: Two parts alcoholic beverage (32 ounces, or 1 L) at 12 percent alcohol combined with 1 part (16 ounces, or 0.5 L) water with 0 percent alcohol gives you a final beverage with 8 percent alcohol. If you use 1 part wine and 1 part water, you would end up with a diluted beverage with 6 percent alcohol, which would also work.

I place the diluted wine (8 percent alcohol) in a jar, then I add my culture (purchased raw vinegar). I like to use around 25 percent of the volume of the wine. So if I have 1 quart (1 L) of diluted wine, I'll add 1 cup (240 ml) of raw vinegar. Once mixed with the diluted wine, the culture will transform the alcohol into acetic acid.

You need oxygen to make vinegar, so cover the jar with a paper towel or clean towel and then secure it with a rubber band or string to protect it from unwanted critters. Now you just need to wait. If all goes well, you'll see a gooey layer forming on top of the liquid within 3 to 4 weeks. That's the mother of vinegar forming! I like to leave my vinegar alone for 4 to 6 weeks, letting the vinegar mother grow as big as ½ inch (1.3 cm) thick.

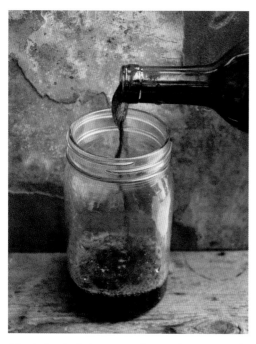

Check the alcohol content of your wine and pour it into a clean jar. If your wine is 12 percent alcohol, fill half the jar.

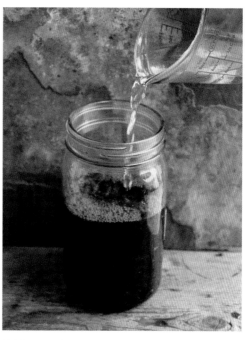

Add ¼ jar of water to dilute the wine. You now have an alcoholic beverage with 8 percent alcohol.

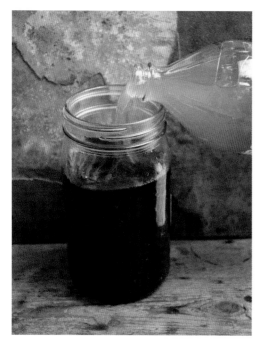

Add around ¼ jar of unpasteurized raw vinegar. You're done!

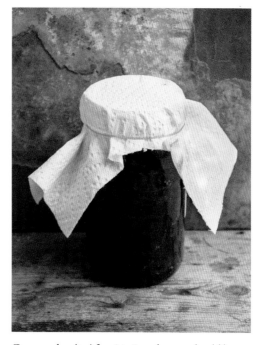

Cover and wait. After 4 to 6 weeks, you should have a mother forming on top. Congratulations! You did it!

Then I strain and bottle the contents. This method is pretty much 100 percent effective.

Keep the mother and some of the new vinegar (see "Storing Your Mother of Vinegar," page 26) for when you'll need it to make more (Using Your Homemade Vinegar Starter).

In summary, these are the ingredients you'll need to make a quart (1 L) jar of vinegar:

2 cups (480 ml) wine (12 percent alcohol)
1 cup water (240 ml)
Around ¾ cup (180 ml) raw vinegar or more (1 cup [240 ml] would work, too)

If you don't have a mother of vinegar after 4 to 6 weeks, something went wrong. There are a number of reasons why it could fail: The culture in the original raw vinegar wasn't alive, the temperature was too cold or too hot, you forgot to dilute the wine, or the vinegar gods just had a bad day. Toss it, and try again with a new raw vinegar. Conversely, during the high-temperature days of summer I've had instances of mothers forming within a couple of weeks.

White Wine and Sparkling Wine

I've had a few failures with store-bought white wine and sparkling wine, particularly white wine. I did some research on this and found I'm not the only one having issues. One reason cited is the lack of tannin and presence of sulfites in white wine. But many of the commercial red wines I use to make vinegars also contain sulfites, so I'm not sure that's the issue.

My solution has been to use organic wine without added chemicals. Furthermore, instead of using a ratio of 80 percent diluted wine to 20 percent raw vinegar, I use 60 percent white wine that's diluted to 8 percent alcohol by volume (ABV) and 40 percent raw vinegar. The first time you do this, you may need to use store-bought raw apple cider vinegar as the starter. You will therefore end up with a blend of white wine and cider vinegar for that first batch. But if you save the resulting vinegar to create more white wine vinegar, you will eventually end up with a pure white wine vinegar. The exact same procedure would apply to sparkling wine.

That said, one of the cheapest white wines at a local supermarket worked beautifully for me, and I've never had an issue making vinegar with it using the regular method of just adding 20 percent raw vinegar. Feel free to try some store-bought white wine and, if you run into a problem, try the approach explained here.

METHOD 2: RAW FERMENTATION: APPLE SCRAPS VINEGAR

Another method for making vinegar at home is raw fermentation—no need to go to the store to get a culture. You can do this with simple alcoholic ferments such as tepache (fermented pineapple), prickly pear wine, or a pear- or apple-scrap ferment, as used in the following process.

The yeast is already present on the ingredients and nothing is boiled, so, with the addition of some sugar, fermentation is assured.

First, the sugar will be converted to alcohol by the wild yeast. You don't want to add too much sugar, as you want your drink to end up in the range of 5 to 9 percent alcohol, which is perfect for the *Acetobacter* bacteria to thrive. The more sugar you add, the higher the alcohol content you will get.

Acetobacter are also present on the fruit scraps. Once your initial alcoholic fermentation is complete, the bacteria will take over and convert the alcohol into vinegar.

Making vinegar with apples is easy. Chop the apples or, if you used the apples for something else, like a pie, and have a lot of scraps left over, you can use those, too. In the old days, throwing away food scraps was frowned upon, and making vinegar was one way to convert scraps into something usable in the kitchen.

Three chopped apples are enough for a quart jar. You want organic, unwaxed apples, if possible, so the yeast is present on the skin. Discard the seeds.

Use the following for a quart (1 L) jar:

> 11 ounces (308 g) apple scraps or chopped apples
> 2 ounces (56 ml) maple syrup or honey or ¼ cup (50 g) sugar
> 2 cups (480 ml) water
> 2 mugwort leaves for flavoring (optional)
> 1 sprig of black sage (*Salvia mellifera*) for flavoring (optional)

Place the apple chunks or scraps in the jar, then add the maple syrup or honey and water.

Add the mugwort leaves and black sage sprig, if using. Once the jar is full, you have two ways to continue the process: open fermentation or anaerobic alcoholic fermentation.

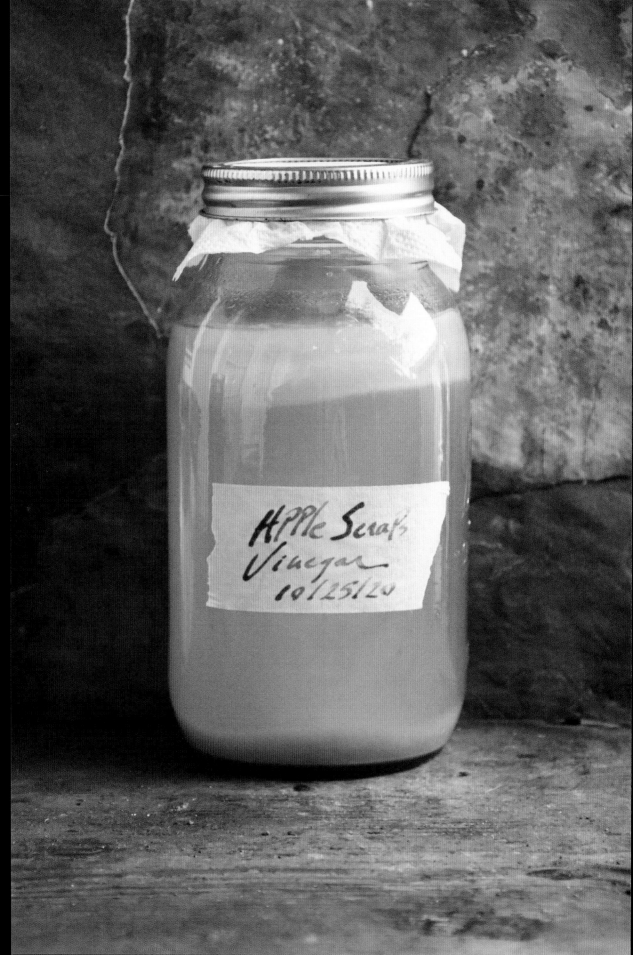

Open Fermentation

Open fermentation is a very traditional method. Secure a dish towel or paper towel on top of the jar with a string or rubber band. At least once a day, remove the towel and stir the contents with a clean spoon for a few seconds, then secure the towel once again. Personally, I stir at least twice a day.

Let me explain the potential problem with this way of fermenting, as well as the solution. Alcoholic fermentation—the first part of the vinegar-making process, before the *Acetobacter* get to work—is usually an anaerobic process, which means it occurs in the absence of oxygen. Mold spores and bacteria that could spoil the food *love* oxygen. Those apple scraps or chunks will float and come into contact with air, meaning unwanted bacteria or mold spores present on the fruit or in the air can proliferate. In other words, you risk mold and spoilage using this method.

The solution is to stir, stir, and stir some more—at least 2 or 3 times daily. The undesirable bacteria and mold spores don't like an acidic environment, which is exactly what's being created with an alcoholic fermentation. As the wild yeast converts the sugar into alcohol, the liquid becomes more acidic, which reduces the chance of spoilage. By stirring daily, you are making sure that all of the jar's contents become acidic, including the floating chunks of fruit. Forget to do it and you're pretty much guaranteed to have mold or other issues on top. Mold is never acceptable, so if your ferment gets moldy, simply toss the mixture and learn from the mistake. Ferment at room temperature (70°F to 80°F [21°C–26°C]) for around 7 to 10 days, then strain out the apple chunks. You should now be able to fit the fermenting liquid in a pint (480 ml) jar.

Cover the top of the pint jar with a dish towel or paper towel and continue the fermentation process. The contents are already quite acidic, but keep stirring at least once a day. Depending on the temperature, the contents will smell like vinegar and have the usual vinegary flavor within a total of 4 to 6 weeks.

Note that you can also stop stirring after you strain out the apple chunks and cover the new jar. It may be a bit riskier, but if you do that, you'll see a mother appear on top after 4 to 6 weeks, which is another indication that your liquid is turning into vinegar. At around 6 weeks, strain and store the mother (see "Storing Your Mother of Vinegar," page 26) and bottle the vinegar.

Anaerobic Alcoholic Fermentation

The second method is to do the initial alcoholic fermentation in an anaerobic environment. If you make a lot of ferments, like I do, then you probably

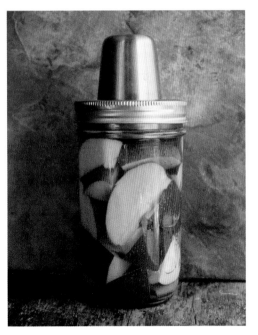

Place all your ingredients in a jar and cover with a clean dish towel, a lid and top, or an airlock.

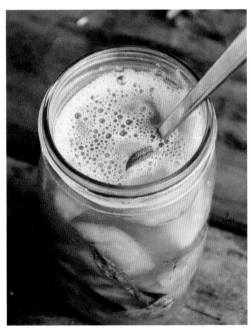

Stir or shake the contents twice (or more) daily. If you used a regular lid and top, you'll need to "burp" the ferment as necessary.

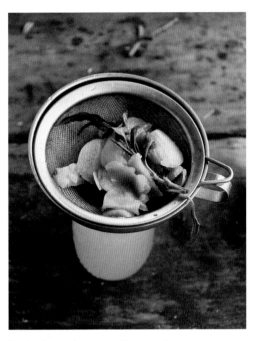

Strain the apple scraps after a week or so.

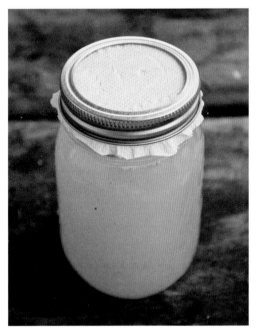

Transfer the liquid into a pint (480 ml) jar and cover with a clean dish towel or paper towel. A mother should appear in 4 to 6 weeks or sooner.

have some airlocks or similar apparatuses at home. It's not a must, but I think you're increasing your chances of success by using one of these devices.

Instead of an airlock, I sometimes use a jar with a regular lid and band. My method is to shake the contents gently at least twice a day, then open the top slightly to let the fermentation gases escape before closing it back. This is what we call "burping the jar." Make sure you don't forget to burp! A lot of pressure can build up inside that jar and create a mess if the top blows off.

If I use an airlock or similar apparatus, I'll do the same, but, obviously, no need for burping.

After 7 to 10 days, strain out the apple chunks and transfer the liquid into a pint (480 ml) jar. Continue as explained in the previous "Open Fermentation" section, with a dish towel or paper towel secured on top of the jar.

Either method, open or anaerobic alcoholic fermentation, will work. If all you have is a dish towel or paper towel, just go ahead and make sure to stir the contents.

METHOD 3: FRUIT FLY VINEGAR

This is probably the most interesting method I've used. It might be "gross" for a lot of people, but it's effective nevertheless.

So, if you have troubles with the prior methods, it's time to get some help from your little friends—fruit flies! Fruit flies, or vinegar flies, love alcohol and yeast, but as explained earlier, they usually have *Acetobacter* as part of their gut microbiota and on their body. This is why wine and beer makers are scared of fruit flies—they can infect their brew or wine and turn it to vinegar.

Southern California is loaded with fruit flies; maybe you have them where you live, too. My method is to pour wine into a jar and dilute it with water in order to obtain 6 to 8 percent alcohol by volume, then leave the jar outside and let the flies find it.

You can even place a sign near the jar that says "Free Wine," so the flies can see it. It doesn't take long—within a few hours you'll have a pool party going on in the jar. Some of the flies may be floating on top of the alcoholic beverage, while others will be on the surface of the glass above the liquid.

Quickly cover the jar with a paper towel, screw the band, and shake the jar gently. That's all you need to do. For a three-quarters-full pint jar, you're looking for 10 to 20 flies.

A vinegar mother will usually start forming on top within 3 weeks. I like to wait 4 to 6 weeks before collecting it. No need for the dead fruit flies anymore—you can toss the wine vinegar that was created and keep the mother.

Use the mother of vinegar as a starter (Using Your Homemade Vinegar Starter) to make vinegar from new alcoholic beverages.

If you have problems attracting fruit flies, place apple or pear scraps on a plate inside a plastic bag and leave the bag somewhat open. Wait until you have a bunch of fruit flies inside, which can take a few days, then place another plastic bag on top of the opening and shake the original plastic bag (with the scraps) until you see them flying into the new one.

Secure the new plastic bag containing the fruit flies on top of the jar containing the alcoholic beverage. Slowly remove the air and tap on the bag so the flies fall into the beverage.

Don't think too much with this method! Get fruit flies inside your jar by whatever means, then cover the jar and wait until you see a mother forming on top. Let it age for a while so the vinegar mother is at least ¼ inch (0.6 cm) thick, then take that mother and use it to make new vinegar with clean wine, beer, mead, and so forth.

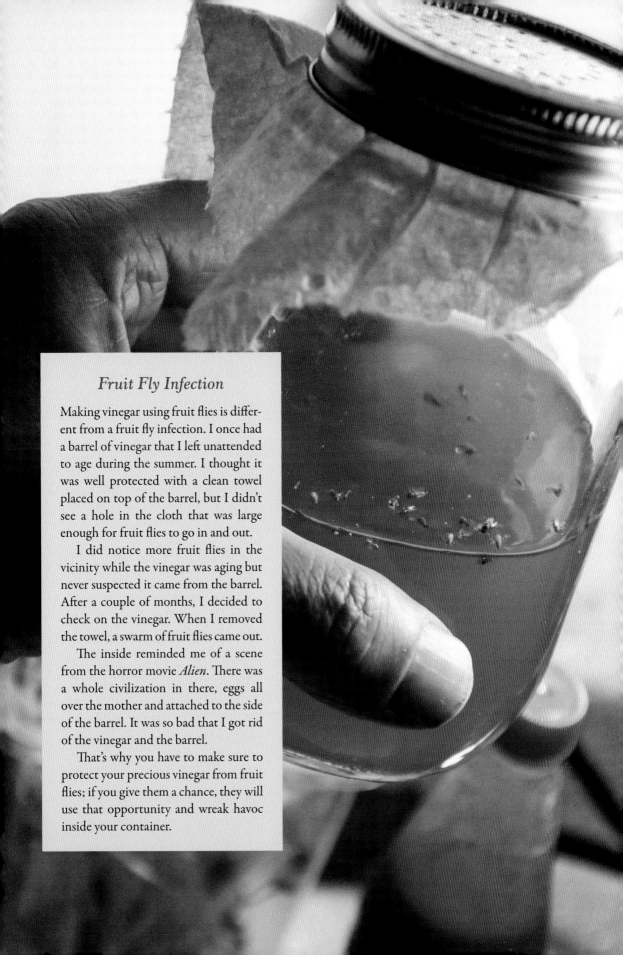

Fruit Fly Infection

Making vinegar using fruit flies is different from a fruit fly infection. I once had a barrel of vinegar that I left unattended to age during the summer. I thought it was well protected with a clean towel placed on top of the barrel, but I didn't see a hole in the cloth that was large enough for fruit flies to go in and out.

I did notice more fruit flies in the vicinity while the vinegar was aging but never suspected it came from the barrel. After a couple of months, I decided to check on the vinegar. When I removed the towel, a swarm of fruit flies came out.

The inside reminded me of a scene from the horror movie *Alien*. There was a whole civilization in there, eggs all over the mother and attached to the side of the barrel. It was so bad that I got rid of the vinegar and the barrel.

That's why you have to make sure to protect your precious vinegar from fruit flies; if you give them a chance, they will use that opportunity and wreak havoc inside your container.

The Mother of Vinegar

The gelatinous, jellyfish-like substance that forms on top of an alcoholic beverage turning to vinegar is called a mother of vinegar, or MOV. It's composed of cellulose and acetic acid bacteria (*Acetobacter*) that develop during the fermentation process.

If you disturb a vinegar that has a mother on top, either by displacing the container or shaking it somehow, the mother may sink to the bottom of the container and a new one will form again on top. It's not a big deal and it doesn't ruin anything. There is no need to keep too many mothers in your vinegar, though. I usually remove the sunken mother right away and use it to make more vinegar, or I store it in the fridge.

Think of the mother of vinegar culture as a starter that can be added to wine, beer, cider, or other alcoholic liquids to turn them into vinegar. If you're into making kombucha, you'll recognize that a mother of vinegar looks very similar to a SCOBY (symbiotic culture of bacteria and yeast). Sometimes people confuse the two, but the culture content is slightly different.

You're pretty much guaranteed to have success in your vinegar-making activities once you have a nice mother of vinegar packed with vinegar bacteria. It's totally possible to make more vinegar without a mother if you have some unpasteurized vinegar with live bacteria in it. But by making a vinegar starter using the raw fermentation method or the fruit fly method you can create your own MOV.

Storing Your Mother of Vinegar

If you don't intend to make new vinegar right away or if you have too much of the culture, you can store your mother for future use.

Simply place the mother of vinegar into a jar or similar container and pour enough vinegar over it to cover it. It doesn't matter if you use home-made vinegar or commercial vinegar, either will keep the culture alive.

Close the container or jar. At this point the fermentation process is already done and you don't need any oxygen. In fact, leaving the container open could be detrimental to the culture, as doing so can cause the acidity of the vinegar to decrease over time. It's also a good idea to choose the right size jar or container so you don't have too much oxygen in it. Don't store your vinegar in a quart jar if it's only one-quarter full—use a pint jar instead.

When I lived in the hot Southern California climate, I personally stored my mother of vinegar in the fridge. It's not a must—you can store it at room temperature, around 68°F (20°C), preferably in a somewhat

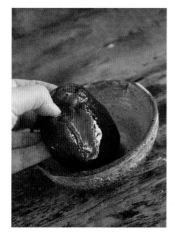

Red wine vinegar mother.

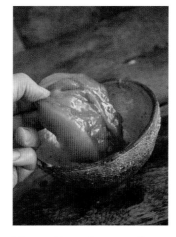

Mugwort beer vinegar mother.

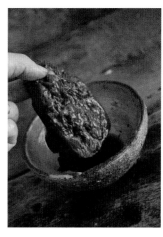

Elderberry wine vinegar mother.

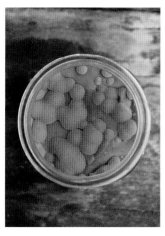

Pomegranate wine vinegar mother.

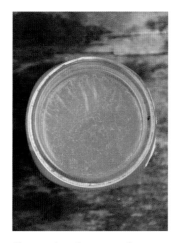

Guava wine vinegar mother.

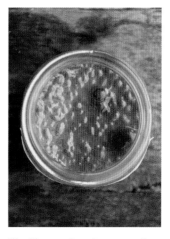

Blackberry wine vinegar mother.

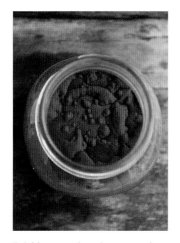

Prickly pear wine vinegar mother.

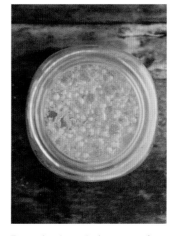

Pear wine (perry) vinegar mother.

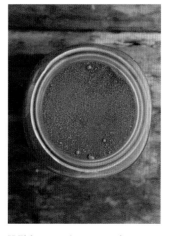

Wild grape vinegar mother.

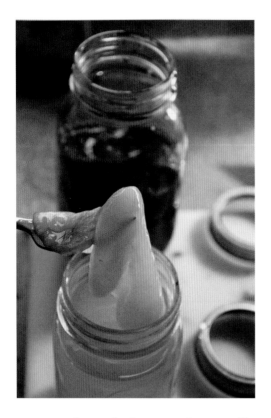

dark place such as inside a cabinet or the basement.

I tend to use the mothers I've stored within a couple of months, but some people say the culture can stay alive for many more months, even years. I've never verified those claims. Around 2 months works perfectly.

The Beauty of Wild Mothers

Fermenting a drink using wild yeast and letting it turn naturally into vinegar creates an incredible array of textures and colors that I've never been able to achieve by introducing a store-bought culture. For example, my pomegranate and prickly pear wines generate mothers that look like creatures from another universe. True beauty. This is probably due to the diversity of yeast and bacteria that can be found in the wild.

If you adventure into wild fermentation and let nature turn your boozy concoctions into vinegar, don't expect your mothers to look like typical mothers. Nature is an amazing artist. Mothers can have a jaw-dropping diversity in their appearances.

So don't freak out. You just need to learn to recognize the differences between mold, an unusual mother forming, and a Kahm yeast film.

Kahm yeast is a common occurrence in home fermentation. It forms a thin whitish layer on the top of the ferment, sometimes creating air bubbles underneath. It often has a stringy look to it, like a spider web. I think it smells cheesy, too. Kahm yeast is not toxic but will influence the flavors of your vinegar in a negative way. I invite you to use an internet search engine and look at photos of Kahm yeast. It pays to know what you're looking at. For example, my guava wine mother nearly looked like Kahm yeast. But the mother was gelatinous, so I knew it was just unusual rather than problematic.

Mold can appear in all kinds of colors, from white to blue, green, red, and so on. It has a fuzzy or hairy surface, while a mother of vinegar is smoother and more gelatinous.

I'm a big fan of food safety, and mold is never acceptable in my world. If I have mold, I toss the ferment. So far it hasn't happened with my vinegars.

Storing Your Vinegar

Aging and properly storing your vinegar is important, and they will influence its flavors. When it is young, vinegar has a sharp bite; this will mellow over time.

A lot of websites and books will tell you that vinegar, because of its high acidity, can keep indefinitely. It's kind of true, but at the same time it isn't. I think it's probably true for white vinegar, which I find tasteless. But a delicious homemade vinegar, if it isn't stored properly, will eventually lose flavor through evaporation and may develop a cloudy appearance.

If you think about it, an elderberry wine vinegar or a smoked mushroom–infused vinegar does have components other than acetic acid; otherwise, it would simply taste like a regular white vinegar. While vinegar itself (acetic acid and water) has an extremely long shelf life, the other components can degrade over time. If you don't store your vinegar properly, you may end up with a murky, flavorless, acidic liquid. And who wants to use that?

Note that we're not talking weeks or months for this type of degradation—it's often years. However, I did have some raw blackberry-infused vinegar with an improperly screwed top that didn't look too good after 7 or 8 months. It was cloudy, had some sediment at the bottom, and underwent a definite degradation in terms of flavor. I'm confident it was not harmful to consume, but it wasn't a fantastic vinegar at that stage.

So yes, you need to properly store your homemade vinegar or it can go "bad" in terms of aesthetics and flavors.

Here are the basic guidelines I follow when storing my vinegars:

- Store it in a proper container. Don't use anything made of copper, brass, iron, and the like, as they will corrode. When I participated in the Master Food Preserver classes through the University of California extension programs, we were told that glass, plastic, wood, enamel, or stainless-steel containers could be used for making or storing vinegar. My humble opinion is that it's best to stick with glass containers.
- For longer shelf life, fill the bottle as much as possible to remove excess oxygen. Close the lid tightly and avoid opening unnecessarily.
- Store your containers in a somewhat cool and dark place. As my climate is quite hot, I store my herb- and fruit-infused vinegars in the fridge.
- While it is true that properly stored vinegar will last indefinitely, not all experts agree. Some argue that, for optimum flavors, homemade vinegars should be consumed within 2 to 3 years. Some even go lower (6 months). I think 2 to 3 years is a good rule.

USING YOUR HOMEMADE
VINEGAR STARTER

This process is pretty much identical to Method 1: Using Unpasteurized Vinegar as a Starter. The main difference is that by using a homemade starter you'll have a much higher success rate. You also won't have the issue of a possible failure because your store-bought vinegar wasn't alive anymore.

Using a homemade starter is also a good way to go if you don't want to mix vinegars. For example, if I decide to make vinegar from my elderberry wine, I would rather use an elderberry wine culture than purchased raw apple cider or red wine vinegar. The flavors dilute too much if you add a somewhat large volume of a different kind of vinegar and mother as a starter.

Ingredients for a 1-quart jar (1 L)
1½ cups (360 ml) wine
1½ cups (360 ml) water
¾ cup (180 ml) mother and live vinegar

Procedure
1. Purchase a bottle of red wine. I usually don't buy an expensive wine to make vinegar, but it's really up to you. You can also use a homemade wine.
2. Look at the label to determine the wine's alcohol by volume (ABV). You will need to dilute your wine so it is between 3 and 9 percent alcohol, as described in the following steps.
3. Let's say you are using a wine that is 13 percent alcohol, for example. Pour 1½ cups (360 ml) of that wine into a quart (1 L) jar.
4. Add 1½ cups (360 ml) water to the wine so the resulting liquid is diluted by 50 percent and has an alcoholic content of 6.5 percent. At this point your jar will

be three-quarters full. The remaining space will be for your starter.
5. Get a fresh mother of vinegar from another jar or a mother that has been preserved.
6. Add the mother of vinegar to your new jar. There is no real rule as to how much mother you should use. If I want to make a bunch of vinegars from some of my wildcrafted wines or beers and I have a limited number of mothers, I may cut them in two or three pieces.
7. Pour some of the live vinegar from your starter jar into the new jar of diluted red wine. As for the amount of live vinegar, I tend to add around 20 percent of the diluted wine volume, about ⅔ cup (144 ml) in this case.
8. Place a clean dish towel or paper towel on top and secure it with a rubber band, string, or lid band.
9. At around 6 weeks, strain and store the mother, which can be used as a future starter. Then bottle the vinegar.

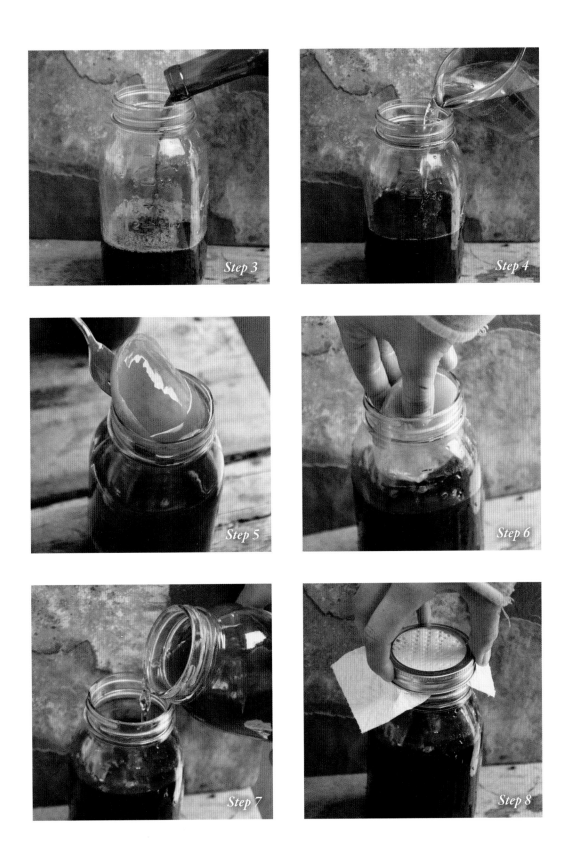

Step 3

Step 4

Step 5

Step 6

Step 7

Step 8

Pasteurizing Your Vinegar

Most of the vinegars you purchase at the store are pasteurized, and you have the option of doing so, too, with your homemade vinegar. There are pro and cons for pasteurizing your homemade vinegar.

Pasteurizing will kill any live bacteria present in the vinegar and stop the fermentation process, thus making your vinegar more stable. You don't run the risk of a mother forming inside your container and creating aesthetic issues. This is probably the main reason commercial vinegars are pasteurized—it looks more appealing for customers when the liquid is transparent, crisp, and free of cloudiness.

However, pasteurizing eliminates the vinegar's probiotic qualities and changes its flavors somewhat. But once the pasteurization is finished, the flavors will stay quite stable indefinitely. I'm still enjoying pasteurized mead vinegar I made 7 years ago and I've never noticed a change in taste.

If you like to give vinegars as gifts, it may also be a good idea to pasteurize it, as you can't control how people will store their vinegar and when they'll use it.

I'll be honest, I don't pasteurize my vinegars anymore and they're always used within a year or two. I think a bit of cloudiness in a raw vinegar shows that it's a good-quality product.

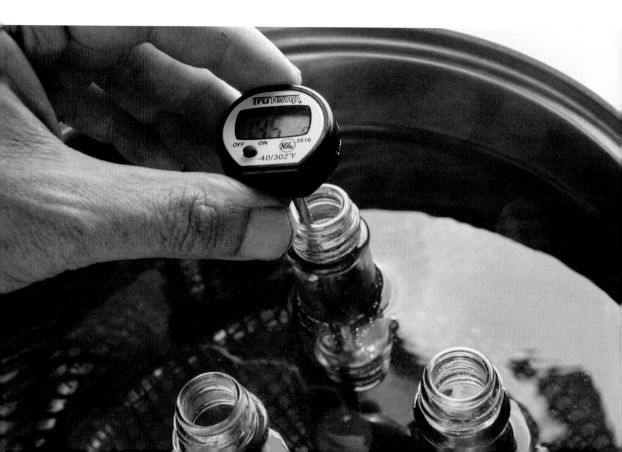

But if you want to pasteurize, the method is quite straightforward. Bottle your vinegar, leaving the caps off, and place the bottles in a water bath canner (or similar setup). Bring the temperature of the vinegar to at least 140°F (60°C) and no more than 160°F (70°C) and cap. Another option is to heat your vinegar to these same temperatures prior to bottling, then pour the liquid into sterilized bottles while it is still hot. Cap the bottles and you're done.

A little tip: After capping the bottles, I immediately place the bottles upside down for 4 to 5 minutes to "pasteurize" the cap.

Determining Acidity

For most vinegars I create, I don't care too much about their precise acidity, as I use them to create drinks, sauces, quick pickles, salad dressings, and for other culinary uses. But if you intend to use a preservation method such as water bath canning (see "Water Bath Canning," page 236), then knowing the acidity is more important.

The FDA considers a vinegar acceptable to use in home canning if it has a strength of 5 percent or higher. Many existing pickling and water bath canning recipes found online, in books, or in other sources have been tested for food safety and use a vinegar with at least 5 percent acidity. If you use a weaker vinegar, you alter the recipe and, from the FDA perspective, the end product may not be acidic enough to prevent spoiling in the long run. This is particularly important in industrial or home canning due to the possibility of botulism, a deadly toxin that can occur in improperly canned products with a pH of 4.6 or above (note that a higher pH means a lower acidity). Consider investing in a good pH meter (for details, see "Checking the pH," page 178).

For the longest time I struggled with the question of how to determine the acidity of my vinegar. There is a scientific technique called acid–base titration, but it's a bit complex for an average person like me.

In titration, a basic solution (pH > 7) of known concentration is used to determine the acid concentration of an unknown solution. Based on the reaction, you can extrapolate the amount of acid in the unknown solution.

For example, to determine the amount of acetic acid in vinegar, the acetic acid will be titrated with a solution of a known concentration of sodium hydroxide (lye, or caustic soda). The reaction can be made visible using a chemical indicator whose color depends on the acid–base ratio. The usual indicator used is a compound known as phenolphthalein. From there, you can calculate the concentration of the acetic acid in your vinegar.

So, in somewhat plain English, you add a solution with a specific amount of lye or caustic soda to a vinegar, then based on the color of the indicator you'll make some calculations and determine acidity. Something like that....

There are plenty of tutorials and videos online that explain the process. Another solution is to test the pH of the preserves before serving them, but most people don't have the tools to do that (lye, a digital pH meter, or pH strips). On the positive side, there are other ways, albeit less precise, to get a good approximation of your vinegar's acidity percentage without those materials.

If you know the amount of alcohol in the liquid you're about to turn into vinegar, you can figure out the approximate acidity of the final product. It's easy to do if you make vinegar from a commercial alcoholic beverage such as wine or beer, as the information about alcohol content can be found on the label.

In theory, a beverage with 8 percent alcohol should give you a vinegar with 8 percent acidity. I'm sure you're thinking, "Dang, that's simple!" But don't get too excited yet.

It's a bit different in practice, as there are several factors that will change the outcome. Some alcohol will evaporate during the vinegar-making process, wild *Acetobacter* don't always behave in the same way as specific commercial strains, and you also have to contend with environmental factors such as temperature, storage, and what the vinegar gods think of your project.

In view of all that, you can expect that a beverage with 8 percent alcohol will convert to a vinegar with 6.4 percent acidity or a bit more. In other words, you lose around 20 percent of the potential acidity in the conversion process. That's good news though, because based on that information, you can dilute an alcoholic beverage to 7 percent alcohol and turn it into a vinegar that will have around 5.6 percent acetic acid by volume. This is why I mostly ferment with an alcoholic beverage that is around 7 or 8 percent alcohol by volume. I know that, in the end, I'll end up with a vinegar that's between 5 and 6 percent acidity.

The other solution is to ferment a beverage with a specific amount of sugar, knowing that the result will be an alcoholic beverage with 7 percent alcohol (see "Determining Sugar Content and Potential Alcohol," page 51, for ratios). If you're an experienced brewer, you can be even more precise and use a hydrometer to calculate the exact amount of alcohol you achieved.

If you want a cute mathematical equation, it looks like this:

10% alcohol by volume × 0.8 = 8% acetic acid by volume

Again, unless you intend to do some canning, I don't think it's that important to know exactly how acidic your vinegar is. In the culinary industry, and from the FDA's perspective, a vinegar should contain 5 to 8 percent acetic acid by volume; but factually, you can make homemade vinegar with a lower or higher amount of acetic acid. Most commercial vinegars start with a high amount of acetic acid and are diluted with water to 5 percent acidity by volume before they are sold.

Personally, I have canned wild edibles with homemade vinegars, but I have a lot of experience with canning, studied food safety, and understand the principles behind it. I also take the precaution of calculating the pH of my recipes before canning and before serving if I have any doubts. If you don't have much experience with canning or food safety issues, stick to a commercial vinegar with 5 percent acidity.

Making Vinegar in a Barrel

I currently make most of my vinegars in regular jars, but in the past I've also used vinegar barrels. They're quite awesome. I can't use them at present because of my traveling lifestyle, but as you'll see later on in this book, other options exist for exploring woody flavors when making vinegar.

There are a few companies that sell vinegar barrels. They are available in various designs and volumes. If you're interested, a simple online search for "vinegar barrels" will provide you with links to these companies. These barrels are usually made of oak, which adds tannin—a naturally occurring astringent substance that helps the fermentation. Most of these barrels have an open top, which must be covered with a clean towel or similar to prevent fruit flies and other critters from infecting the precious vinegar. Some barrels come with a top or "cork." You typically have the option of ordering the barrels toasted or untoasted.

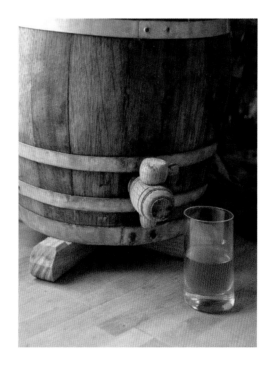

I like to use the toasted barrels for red and wild berry wines. I prefer untoasted barrels for simple vinegars like Method 2: Raw Fermentation: Apple Scraps Vinegar and my wild beers, but there are no rules. It's all about your own taste buds. I've even had good success making white wine vinegar (which can be finicky) in wooden barrels.

Once you receive the barrel, you'll need to prep it by rinsing the inside with water a couple of times. You can use boiling water to kill any unwanted bacteria. Next, you tap the spigot into place with a mallet, then fill 90 percent of the barrel with water. In the beginning it may drip a little and you will need to add water, but by the next day, the dripping should stop as the wood swells. Empty the water and you're ready to go. One of my barrels didn't seal properly due to a factory defect, but I fixed it by using an old Belgian trick of applying wet dough paste to the problem area on the outside of the barrel. There are many other methods for sealing the leaks of an oak barrel, and you can find how-to instructions online.

Whether you purchase a regular oak barrel or a toasted one, your first batch of vinegar using a barrel might have too much bitter oak or smoky flavor if you age it too long. I had that problem with my first red wine vinegar in a toasted barrel. My solution was to dilute the finished product with regular red wine vinegar until I was satisfied with the taste.

When I purchased a new toasted barrel, I filled it with a good commercial apple cider vinegar and let it sit for a couple of weeks. That vinegar turned out delicious. Then I proceeded to use the barrel to make my homemade vinegars.

To make homemade vinegar in a barrel, use the same ratio of wine to raw vinegar as you would with a jar. Fill the barrel with around 80 percent diluted wine and 20 percent raw vinegar. Leave around 2 inches (5 cm) headspace and cover with a clean towel.

Keep your barrel in a shaded and ventilated area with an ambient temperature of 70 to 85°F (21–30°C). In approximately 6 to 8 weeks, the vinegar should be ready with a beautiful mother on top. If you decide to age the vinegar for a longer period, check the flavor from time to time.

Technically, after that first fermentation you could empty the barrel and simply add diluted wine to make more vinegar. The fermentation would take off, as *Acetobacter* will already be present in the wood from the previous bath. But, to play it safe, I always leave around 25 percent of the vinegar with some mother in the barrel, and then I add new diluted wine.

Some people do things a bit differently—they'll leave 50 percent of the vinegar and just add undiluted wine. Instead of water, the vinegar itself dilutes the wine. Makes sense.

Continuous Fermentation

I remember visiting a restaurant in Belgium as a teenager. The chef had a barrel in the kitchen into which he would pour the leftovers from red wine bottles he used for cooking or nearly emptied bottles he could not serve to his customers. It didn't really matter if it was a Bordeaux or Cabernet Sauvignon, he would simply pour the contents into the barrel without adding any water for dilution. The barrel was pretty much always three-quarters full of vinegar, so diluting wasn't an issue.

I think this practice was quite normal in the old days. Food waste was frowned upon, and having a constant supply of vinegar that tasted better than commercial red wine vinegar was a big plus. This was true for restaurants, and also for regular households or farmhouses. Going to the store before cars were introduced wasn't that easy, and it was important to be self-reliant.

The concept of a continuous fermentation makes sense. There are all kinds of variations, but the basic logic is that if a barrel is mostly full of vinegar, then any small amount of wine added will ferment quite quickly.

Most of the work involves starting the initial fermentation, exactly as explained in "Making Vinegar in a Barrel," page 35. Fill the barrel with around 80 percent diluted wine and 20 percent raw vinegar. Leave around 2 inches (5 cm) headspace and cover with a clean towel.

Keep your barrel in a shaded and ventilated area with an ambient temperature of 70 to 85°F (21–30°C). In approximately 6 to 8 weeks the fermentation should be complete.

You're now ready to start fermenting more vinegar. Remove around 25 percent of the vinegar and store it. Save and store the mother if you want to start other ferments.

From there, the methods will vary a bit. A chef in a restaurant will use a lot of vinegar and have a decent supply of leftover wines. In the old days, it didn't really matter if the vinegar still had some alcohol in it. For a French or Belgian chef it was *vin aigre*, which means "sour wine." They really didn't think much about it: Vinegar was used as needed and wine was added as it was available. I call it the "in and out" method.

French cuisine is full of recipes using vinegar for cooking, sauces, salad dressings, and preservation. If the vinegar was used for cooking or creating

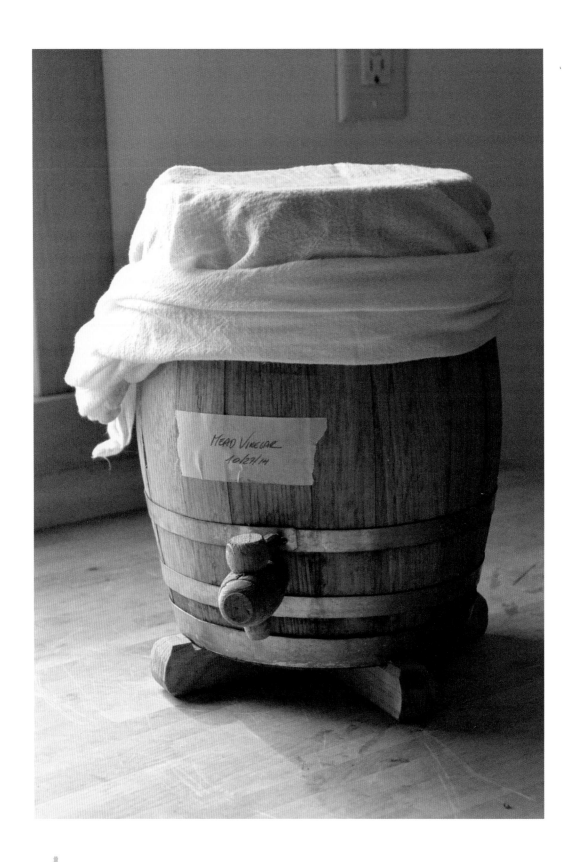

The handwritten label on the barrel reads: "MEAD VINEGAR 10/29/14"

sauces, whatever small amount of alcohol was in it would simply evaporate during the process.

Yes, it was crude, but it worked. One of the French chefs I worked with in Los Angeles used that method with success. To be honest, it was a bit intuitive. The chef would taste the vinegar as part of his daily routine and if he felt there was too much alcohol or it needed aging, he would simply take the appropriate actions. If the barrel was too full, he would bottle the excess vinegar and store it.

Later on, this chef even added a couple more barrels so he could decide to age one of the barrels for a few months if he wanted to and work with the other two in the meantime. One barrel was used for white wine vinegar.

That's the advantage of working closely with your ferments; you are in control and make decisions based on actual flavors. If you feel there is too much alcohol, just let the vinegar ferment for a couple of weeks. If you think the vinegar needs a bit of aging to mellow the flavors, leave it alone for a while. Simple.

Another method, albeit less intuitive, is to collect a specific amount of vinegar from the original fermentation, bottle it, and replace it with an equal volume of wine.

For example, if your barrel has a volume of 1 gallon (4 L), you can remove 1 quart (1 L) of vinegar. Store and age that vinegar and add 1 quart (1 L) of wine to the barrel. Wait 3 to 4 weeks, taste, and if you like it, repeat the process. If you need to age it more, you can do so.

You can remove as much as 50 percent of the barrel's contents and add 2 quarts (2 L) of red wine. I would suggest you dilute the wine to around 10 percent alcohol, but some people don't dilute it and end up with a strong vinegar. Wait a tad longer than for the 1-quart addition, because you now have more alcohol that needs to ferment. After 4 to 6 weeks, taste and repeat the process.

When I was working with local restaurants, I did a continuous fermentation for 3 years with 4 different barrels that were 1 gallon (4 L) each. One barrel for wild beers, one for red wine, one for wild wines (elderberry, blackberry, and others) and one for white wine. I never experienced any problems.

I must admit I was very loose with the process. It wasn't unusual for me to leave the barrels alone for 3 to 4 months before using some of the vinegar and replacing it with new beer or wine. The mother would be quite large, but I would share it with friends and students.

I think changing the barrel every 2 to 3 years is a good idea. After 3 years I can no longer detect the toasty, woody flavor in the vinegar.

Continuous fermentation is not a complicated process. In fact it's quite easy if you work with your ferment. A wooden barrel is not your only option; you can also use a ceramic water cooler or crock.

Vinegar Eels

Eels in my vinegar?! Don't panic yet! I've made vinegar for over 20 years and I've never seen eels. But apparently it can happen. The first time I heard of vinegar eels, I immediately pictured regular, 3-feet-long eels, and I was so confused! But no, they're super tiny.

Vinegar eels (*Turbatrix aceti*) are tiny animals that feed on the mother of vinegar. They're not related to the eels you find in the ocean or in rivers but are more like worms and are classified along with insects. They are nematodes, which are tiny worms that can be found in countless environments— from sea to fresh water to terrestrial environments. It is estimated that the number of nematode species could reach 1,000,000 or more.

I have not been able to take a photo of the little guys, as I've never had them in my vinegars, but if you search for "vinegar eels" online, you'll find lots of photos. An infection looks like a mass of little worms feeding on the mother.

The good news is that they're not toxic. Based on my research, they can be quite common in industrial vinegar facilities. The FDA doesn't have a problem with them. I quote from their regulation:

Because some information which indicates that vinegar eels aid in vinegar production, we do not believe the finding of vinegar eels in a firm's bulk storage tanks or generators should be considered as an objectionable condition unless the firm's filtration system is not functioning or unless the eels are present in the finished product.

POLICY:

The finding of vinegar eels in finished product would be considered objectionable and would render the finished product adulterated within the meaning of 402(a)(3).*

So there you have it. Vinegar eels are not objectionable in commercial vinegar production as long as they're filtered out and not present in the finished product, which is your store-bought bottle.

The consensus among regular people like us making homemade vinegar is simple—toss the vinegar, thoroughly clean the container or pasteurize it, then restart.

---

* "CPG Sec 525.825 Vinegar, Definitions— Adulteration with Vinegar Eels," US Food and Drug Administration, last updated March 1995, https://www.fda.gov /regulatory-information/search-fda -guidance-documents/cpg-sec-525825 -vinegar-definitions-adulteration -vinegar-eels.

CHAPTER 2

Creating Unique Vinegars

N ow we're entering the rabbit hole. In this chapter we'll explore the diverse possibilities of homemade, wildcrafted vinegars, and believe me, the possibilities are endless.

As I write this book, I have around 36 different wildcrafted vinegars happily fermenting on my shelves. Most of them are derived from alcohol made by wild yeast fermentation. If you want to explore homebrewing and alcoholic fermentation, I have an entire book on the subject, called *The Wildcrafting Brewer*. Making your own homemade alcoholic beverages is not a must but will greatly increase the range of creative possibilities.

To make a unique vinegar, not every ingredient has to be collected from the wild. So in this chapter we'll look at the various ways you can make a unique vinegar with both wildcrafted and store-bought ingredients. The recipes follow the methods we learned about in chapter 1, with some slight variations. But essentially, the process is always either letting a ferment turn into vinegar naturally or introducing a culture starter to a fermented beverage.

There is a huge variety of beverages, ingredients, and liquids that can be turned into homemade vinegar, including the following:

Commercial beers or wines
Distilled spirits
Chopped fruits or scraps
Homemade (wildcrafted)
    meads, beers, and wines

Homemade or store-bought
    fruit juices
Fruit mashes
Custom "brews"

As you'll see in greater detail, you can make unusual brews for the sole purpose of making vinegars with particular flavors. I call them "brews" because they don't quite fit definitions or labels such as beer, wine, or mead. I've made forest and mountain brews with all kinds of plants collected in the wild and fermented with sugar sources such as molasses, maple syrup, and even insect honeydew (lerps sugar). Brews are where you can truly unleash your creativity!

Vinegar from Commercial Beers or Wines

You can create vinegars out of any commercial beer, wine, or spirit. It is very simple to make. You just need to add store-bought unpasteurized vinegar or some that you made at home (see Method 1: Using Unpasteurized Vinegar as a Starter). I'll focus on making vinegars with beer in this section, as method 1 covers what you need to know about making vinegar from wines.

The main problem I've experienced with making vinegar from beer is that cheap, commercial brands don't always do well. I'm not sure why, but I imagine there are probably some preservatives and chemical additives in those beers that vinegar bacteria don't like much. And even when I've had success, the resulting vinegar has been somewhat bland.

Wildcrafted vinegars of all shades.

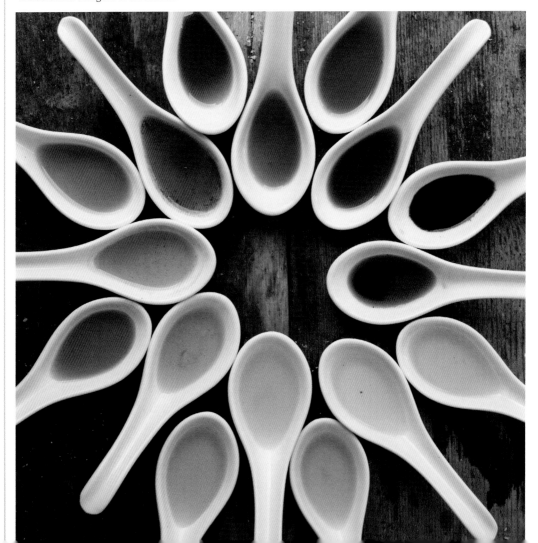

If you want to make terrific beer vinegars, spend a bit of money and go for artisanal and organic beers. You have so many choices! Many hoppy beers have delicious fruity, flowery, and citrusy flavors that translate quite well into vinegar. I'm not a fan of too much hops, but I like fruity beers. I've made some delicious vinegar with *gueuzes*, which are Belgian sour beers made with wild yeast and often flavored with fruits or berries. The last beer vinegar I made was with a beer called Kriek Belle-Vue, which is made by macerating fresh cherries into a sour (lambic) beer, giving the beer a beautiful red color.

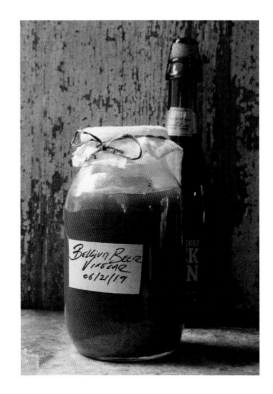

As always, check the label and look at the alcoholic content of the beer. Most beers will be around 5 percent alcohol by volume (ABV), but some beer styles, such as stouts, can have up to 10 percent ABV. You'll have some extremes—beers approaching 20 percent ABV—but those are the exceptions.

I like to use beers with at least 5 percent ABV to make my vinegar. I've had problems with Kahm yeast (see "The Beauty of Wild Mothers," page 28) when using beers with a lower alcohol content.

In the case of my Belgian beer (Kriek Belle-Vue), I simply pour the beer into a quart (1 L) jar, filling it three-quarters of the way, then add my culture, which is either unpasteurized store-bought or homemade vinegar with a bit of mother. The ratio I use is 75 percent beer to around 25 percent unpasteurized vinegar. Basically, I fill the jar but leave around 1 inch (2.5 cm) of headspace.

You need oxygen to make vinegar, so cover the jar with a paper towel or clean dish towel and secure it with a rubber band or string. Within 3 to 4 weeks, you'll see a mother of vinegar forming on top. Wait another couple of weeks, then strain and bottle the contents. Store the mother so you can use it to create more vinegar.

Young vinegar can be quite sharp. I usually age my vinegar for 2 to 3 months or more before using it. Aging will mellow the flavors, but it's not a must.

Once you start experimenting with beer vinegars it's hard to stop. There are so many excellent beers to choose from!

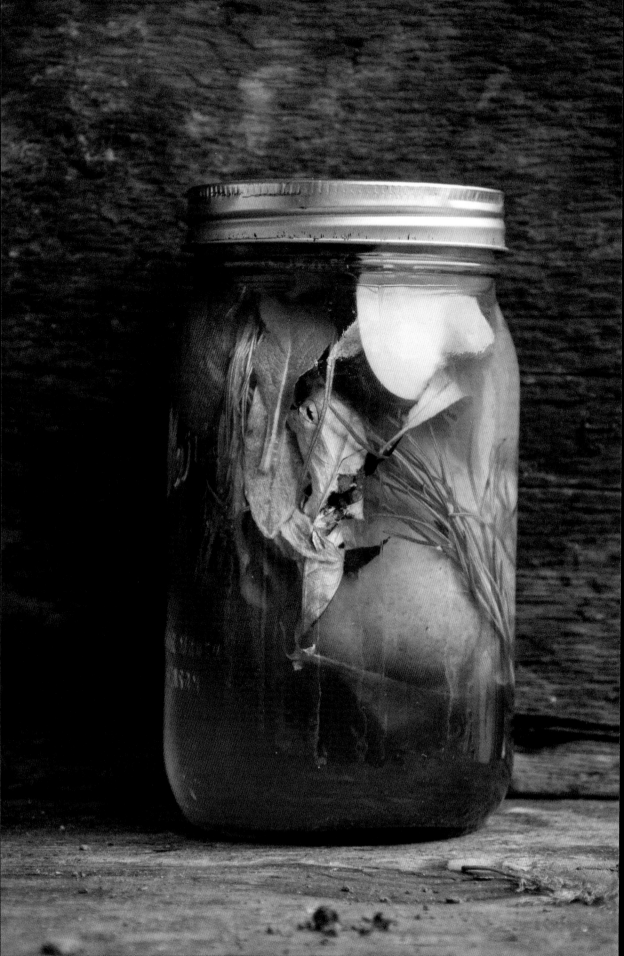

PERRY VINEGAR

Perry is an alcoholic beverage made from fermented pears. It's pretty much identical to cider and uses the same fermentation method. If you like pears, you can make a pear scraps vinegar following the recipe for Method 2: Raw Fermentation: Apple Scraps Vinegar, or you can use whole pears, like I do, and cut them into chunks.

Personally, I like perry vinegar better than apple cider vinegar. I think it's more floral. It's kind of hard to find perry vinegar commercially, so I end up making it myself.

Of course, I must add a touch of the local terroir to give it some local flavor. Yarrow (one large flower) and a couple of mugwort leaves do the work. Not only are both herbs extremely aromatic, but the background bitterness they provide is quite awesome in both cider and perry.

Procedure

The method I use is simple: I just take a quart (1 L) jar and fill half of it with sliced pears—around 12 ounces (340 g)—then add 2 cups (480 ml) of water, herbs for flavoring, and ⅓ cup (80 ml) maple syrup. I try to leave ½ inch (1.3 cm) of headspace, then screw on the lid.

No need for yeast—as with apples, the yeast is present on the fruit's skin.

I don't use an airlock; I just shake the jar twice a day and burp it as necessary. Let it ferment for around 10 days in the jar, then remove the pears and transfer the boozy liquid into a pint jar (480 ml). Place a clean paper towel on top secured by a lid band or rubber band.

At this point, let nature do its thing. The *Acetobacter* will eventually take over and turn the perry into vinegar in around 4 to 6 weeks. If you don't want to take the risk that your perry doesn't turn into vinegar on its own, you can add around 20 percent by volume of commercial unpasteurized vinegar (such as Bragg) or your own homemade vinegar with some mother. You may need a bigger container, though.

After 6 weeks, strain and bottle the vinegar. Store the mother if you want to use it to create more vinegar. Age the bottled vinegar for 2 to 3 months or more before using it. Aging will mellow the flavors, but it's not a must.

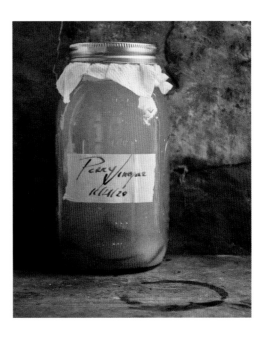

PRICKLY PEAR LAZY WINE VINEGAR

I don't always follow the rules. This ferment is usually more intuitive and based on taste. Normally I don't calculate the amount of sugar I use, but I took note for this book.

I call this kind of wine "lazy wine" because you don't have to do much—just stir the contents from time to time and add sugar to taste until you get the booziness and flavor you're looking for.

One of my favorite methods for making primitive wine is with cactus fruit. These are known as prickly pears (*Opuntia littoralis*). I foraged the fruit from the local coastal prickly pear cactus near where I lived in Southern California. The fruits from the wild cactus are half the size of the ones you can purchase at the store and they contain many more seeds, but I think the flavors are more pronounced. As a wildcrafter, you should forage these fruits at their prime when they're super sweet.

Several methods can be used for harvesting prickly pears. I simply use my bare hands and a small broom, usually one I make with twigs from plants found on location, such as wild mustard or wild oats (*Avena fatua*). I don't use kitchen tongs to remove the prickly pears, burn the glochids (tiny needles) off the fruit, or use any other methods. To remove the needles while the pear is still on the cactus, you just need to vigorously slap or brush the fruit up, down, and sideways for a few seconds, until they are gone. It takes a bit of practice, but it works. Don't do it with the wind blowing toward you or the flying needles will get into your clothes and eventually in your skin.

Once you've removed the glochids, use a hand twist to remove the pears from the cactus plant. Inspect the pears to make sure you got all the glochids, and place them in your bag. Once home, you can rinse them briefly in cold water. Don't use hot water, as it will kill the wild yeast present on the skin.

Ingredients for a ½-gallon jar (2 L)

Around 20 small prickly pears or
   10 larger store-bought prickly pears
4 to 5 ounces (120–140 g) white sugar
Around 1 quart (1 L) water

Procedure

1. Using a knife, stab each prickly pear three or four times, then place them in a clean ½-gallon (2 L) jar. The yeast is already present on the fruits.
2. Add the sugar and the water to the jar. Leave around ½ inch (1.3 cm) of headspace. Close the top or screw the lid on, but not so tightly that fermentation gases cannot escape.

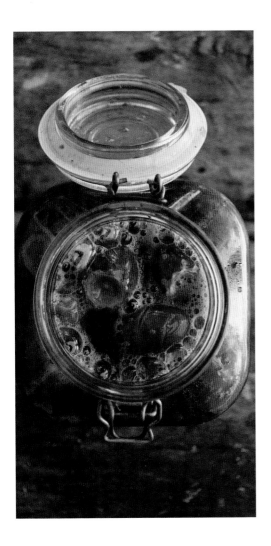

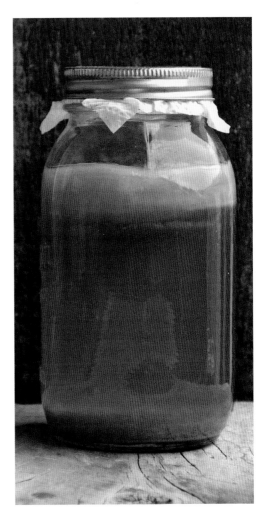

3. With a clean spoon, stir the contents twice daily for 10 seconds or so.

4. After 7 days, taste the ferment. Depending on the temperature (warmer equals faster), the yeast should have converted most of the sugar to alcohol. If it's still quite sweet, continue the fermentation until the liquid is nicely boozy with just a little bit of sweetness.

5. Strain the prickly pears and transfer the liquid to a quart (1 L) jar. Place a clean paper towel on top secured by a lid band or rubber band. At this point I just let nature do its

thing. The *Acetobacter* will take over and turn the wine into vinegar within 4 to 6 weeks. Another option is to add around 20 percent by volume of commercial unpasteurized vinegar (such as Bragg), or your own homemade vinegar with a bit of mother, right after transferring the liquid into the jar. You may need a bigger jar, though.

6. After 6 weeks, strain and bottle the vinegar. Store the mother if you want to use it to create more vinegar. Age the bottled vinegar for 2 to 3 months or more before using it. Aging will mellow the flavors, but it's not a must.

VINEGAR FROM DISTILLED SPIRITS:
12-YEAR-OLD WHISKEY VINEGAR

This was such a fun and interesting project. I'm always a fan of unusual vinegars, and I thought that a good whiskey could make a fantastic product. I'd never heard of a whiskey vinegar and really wanted to try to make some.

Making vinegar from distilled spirits is exactly the same as making vinegar from beers or wines. The only difference is that you'll need to add much more water to dilute the amount of alcohol in the mixture to bring it down to around 7 to 8 percent ABV.

Of course, I wanted to go for the best whiskey, but my budget is kind of small, so I bought a tiny bottle (1 cup, or 240 ml) of 12-year-old whiskey at my local liquor store. Some whiskeys are aged in toasted oak barrels, but this one wasn't, so I decided to add a bit of toasted oak bark to it. I used a kitchen torch and toasted 3 small pieces of bark that were each about ¾ inch (2 cm) long. I transferred the whiskey into a closed jar with the toasted oak bark and aged it for 2 months on my shelf. The end result was delicious: smoky, malty, and not overly acidic.

The following steps are for making vinegar out of whiskey, but you can use any distilled spirit.

Procedure

1. Check the alcohol percentage. My whiskey was 40 percent ABV.
2. Add water to reduce the alcohol percentage. In my case, I had 1 cup (240 ml) of whiskey to start with. I added 4 cups (1 L) of water to reduce the alcohol content to 8 percent. The cool thing about distilled spirits is that a small quantity can be used to make a decent amount of vinegar. I ended up with 5 cups of liquid ready to turn into vinegar.
3. Pour the diluted whiskey (along with the toasted bark if so desired) into a ½-gallon (2-liter) jar.
4. Introduce a starter to initiate the fermentation and turn the diluted whiskey to vinegar. Use either store-bought unpasteurized vinegar or homemade vinegar with some mother. A ratio of 75 percent diluted spirit and around 25 percent culture starter works well. I used 1½ cups (360 ml) of homemade white wine vinegar and mother as a starter for this project.
5. Within 3 to 4 weeks, your vinegar should have a beautiful mother floating on top. Wait another 3 weeks or so, then taste. If it is to your liking, strain and bottle the vinegar. Store the mother if you want to use it to create more vinegar.
6. Age the vinegar for 2 to 3 months or more before using it. Aging will mellow the flavors, but it's not a must.

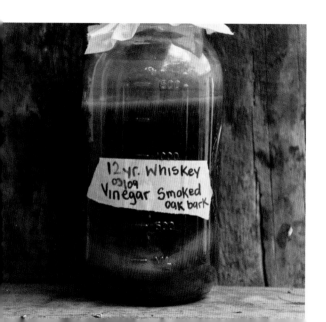

TEPACHE VINEGAR

Tepache is a well-known traditional Mexican fermented drink made from pineapple tops and peels, but you can also use the whole fruit to make tepache. The first step in making tepache vinegar is to create an alcoholic fermentation utilizing the wild yeast already present on the fruit. It's extremely simple to make.

Ingredients for three 1-quart jars (1 L)

1 ripe pineapple
2½ quarts (2.5 L) water
1 piloncillo cone (9 ounces, or 250 g)
    or brown sugar or maple syrup
1 stick cinnamon
3 or 4 cloves
1 dehydrated chili pod (optional,
    but gives a spicy kick to the drink)

Procedure

Chop the pineapple with the peel on. Combine all the ingredients in a large container (glass jar, clay pot, or food-grade bucket).

Cover with a clean towel and stir 3 times daily. The fermentation usually starts on the second day. Strain the pineapple chunks after 4 to 5 days, then pour the liquid back into the container and continue the process.

There are no real rules as to fermentation time. Tepache is usually consumed right away, but you can ferment it for a few more days to get a higher level of alcohol (some people even add beer to it).

To make the vinegar, simply continue the fermentation process with the strained tepache. Keep stirring 3 times daily until eventually the fermentation slows down or stops and you don't have any more fermentation gases (around 10 days, depending on the temperature).

At that point, my method is to simply let nature and the *Acetobacter* already present in the drink do their job. I cover the ferment with a clean towel and leave it alone in a somewhat shady place. Within 4 to 6 weeks, it should have turned to vinegar with a beautiful mother floating on top. Wait another couple of weeks, then strain and bottle the contents. Store the mother if you want to use it to create more vinegar. Age the vinegar for 2 to 3 months or more before using it. Aging will mellow the flavors, but it's not a must.

Another method is to keep stirring the contents daily until the liquid turns into vinegar. The vinegar should be ready a week or so faster with this method, as you oxygenate the contents, but you don't end up with a beautiful mother.

From Creative Yeast Fermentation to Vinegar

At this point, you have several specific recipes for making vinegar from scratch using a homemade alcoholic fermentation. But what if you want to experiment and make your own creative alcoholic ferments without recipes to work from?

If you think about it, the creative potential is quite enormous, as you can create any alcoholic beverage specifically to make vinegar. For example, you could make a wild currant or store-bought Asian pear ferment mixed with lemons, pine needles, and savory or aromatic herbs such as sage, mint, and so on.

With experience, you can truly go deep into local flavors. As you'll see, I've made extremely complex and unique vinegars by brewing ingredients from my local forest, such as mushrooms, barks, roots, and various tasty herbs.

All you need to be successful is enough sugar to create an alcoholic beverage that will give you (with or without dilution) between 5 and 9 percent alcohol content. Technically, you can make a vinegar with a lower amount of alcohol, but in my experience, a low-alcohol ferment can lead to problems such as Kahm yeast or mold.

Some fruits and berries have enough natural sugars that you won't need to add any extra. For example, apple juice normally has enough sugar to make a cider with 5 to 6 percent alcohol, which is perfect if you want to make apple cider vinegar.

Contrast this to blackberries or elderberries, which have enough sugar to create an alcoholic beverage with only 2 to 3 percent alcohol at the most. Thus, when using these fruits you'll need to add sugar so the final fermented drink contains between 5 and 9 percent alcohol.

Grapes can have too much sugar to make vinegar. When you ferment them, you can end up with a wine containing 12 to 13 percent alcohol. In this case, you would need to add water to dilute the juice.

Some ingredients don't have sugar at all. These include hops, yarrow, and mugwort. Therefore, if you want to make vinegar using herbs with no sugar in them, you'll need to add a specific amount of sugar to end up with the necessary alcohol percentage for vinegar making.

And of course, you can also mix ingredients that contain sugar with others that don't have any. I do that all the time with my wild brews, incorporating bitter herbs, fruits, and berries with varying sugar contents.

In summary, to be able to turn your own alcoholic ferment into vinegar, you need to know two things:

1. The attainable alcohol content from the ingredients you collect.
2. How much sugar you need to add, if necessary, to obtain an alcoholic beverage with the right amount of alcohol.

Not everything you might want to ferment will create a pure, translucent juice. For example, the best way to ferment plums is to create a mash by removing the pits, blending or crushing the fruits into a pulp, and adding some water. After fermentation, the mash can be strained, the pulp removed, and the resulting liquid turned into vinegar.

I know it sounds a bit complex, but once you start making vinegar and creating your own recipes, it will become super simple and easy. Start with the recipes in this book to build your confidence and understand how the fermentation process works, then start experimenting.

Realize that you have a decent amount of room for error—a fermented liquid with 5 percent alcohol, 9 percent, or anything in between will be good enough to make vinegar. If you aimed to create a beverage with 7 percent alcohol and you added a bit more sugar than you should have, you could still be all right.

Determining Sugar Content and Potential Alcohol

How do you determine the amount of sugar in your fruit or berries? If they are store-bought, it's quite easy: You'll often find the information related to sugar content on the label. For example, I purchased some blueberries a few days ago. The label on the box said that they contain 0.5 ounce (14 g) of sugar per serving size of 5 ounces (140 g), which means sugar is 10 percent of the weight.

If the packaging of your fruit doesn't list the sugar content, you can go online and do a search for its nutritional data. You'll find several sources with the information you need.

It's quite easy to research the sugar content for commercial fruits and berries, but it can be difficult or even impossible with obscure wild berries. For example, in my local setting I have used manzanita (*Arctostaphylos manzanita*) and coffeeberry (*Frangula californica*). Despite a lot of research, I could not find any information as to their sugar content.

What do you do in such cases?

Personally, I compare them in terms of taste with berries whose sugar content I know. The manzanita berries I collect are not very sweet, similar to a ripe currant berry, so I expect maybe 4 to 5 percent sugar. If it's a bit more or even a bit less, it's still workable. I aim for an alcoholic ferment with 7 percent alcohol, but if it's 6 or 8 percent it will still be all right.

Even experts don't always agree. For example, one publication might list the sugar content for blackberries at 4 to 6 percent, while a website with nutritional information will list the sugar content at 3 to 4 percent. Such variations are due to numerous factors, such as time of harvest, ripeness, location, and so on.

Once you know the sugar content of your fruit, it is quite easy to calculate the potential alcohol you could get by fermenting that fruit. To get your estimate, simply divide the sugar percentage by two.

I've done a lot of research about the sugar content of common wild or store-bought fruits and berries. The results are compiled in table 2.1. Use this information as a rough but helpful guideline. I included rhubarb because we have a lot of related wild plants in Southern California, such as various docks and sorrels. Sugar content is negligible in those plants.

Table 2.1. Percent Sugar and Potential Alcohol of Common Fruits and Berries

Fruit/berry	Sugar (%)	Potential alcohol (%)
Apple	10–14	5–7
Apricot	9–12	5–6
Autumn olive (*Elaeagnus umbellata*)	7–8	3–4
Blackberry	5	2–3
Blueberry (wild)	6.5–8	3–4
Cherry	14	7
Chokeberry (*Aronia melanocarpa*)	4	2
Cranberry	3–4	2
Currant	5–7	2–3
Elderberry	4–5	2–3
Grapes	16–20 (or more)	8–10
Huckleberry	2–3	1
Mulberry	16	8
Orange (navel)	14–15	7–8
Passion fruit	11	5–6
Pear	9–10	5
Pineapple	10	5
Plum	14	7
Pomegranate	14	7
Prickly pear	10–12	5–6
Quince	5	2–3
Raspberry	5	2–3
Rhubarb	1	~
Rose hip (US)	3	1–2
Strawberry	5	2–3

How Much Sugar to Add

Remember that it is a good idea to aim for an alcoholic beverage with 7 percent alcohol or slightly higher. In theory, you should get a vinegar with 7 percent acidity from a beverage with 7 percent alcohol, but in reality, you lose around 20 percent of that potential acidity in the process. So, you should expect a 7 percent alcohol beverage to convert to a vinegar with around 5.6 percent acidity. This is a sort of standard percent in the vinegar industry. It's the amount of acidity you will find in most store-bought vinegars and it's what's recommended by the FDA for canning purposes.

As you can see from table 2.1, if you want to make a prickly pear vinegar, you can simply ferment the juice to get a 5 to 6 percent ABV liquid (a little low, but it will do the trick). You would then let it turn into vinegar on its own (see Method 2: Raw Fermentation: Apple Scraps Vinegar) or add 20 percent unpasteurized vinegar at the end of the alcoholic fermentation, like for making red wine vinegar (see Method 1: Using Unpasteurized Vinegar as a Starter).

But let's say that you want to ferment some blackberry juice. The juice would have enough sugar to create only a 2 to 3 percent alcohol beverage. That's not enough to make vinegar. You need to increase the potential alcohol by 3 or 5 percent to achieve a total of 6 or 7 percent. Table 2.2 indicates the amount of sugar you need to add to 1 quart (1 L) of a liquid to attain a given percentage of alcohol. Following table 2.2, if you have 1 quart (1 L) of blackberry juice, you'll need to add 2.8 ounces (80 g) of sugar to bring the alcohol level up by 4 percent to a total of 6 or 7 percent.

As another example, you might decide to add 25 percent water to your prickly pear juice so it's less thick. But if you do that, you will dilute the amount of sugar in the juice and you may end up with a potential alcohol of between 3.5 to 4 percent. Thus, you'll need to add sugar. In this case you could add 2.1 ounces (60 g) of sugar to bring the potential alcohol to 6.5 or 7 percent.

Table 2.2. Amount of sugar necessary to create a specific amount of alcohol for 1 liter or quart

White/Brown sugar (oz.)	White/Brown sugar (g)	Alcohol obtained (%)
0.7	20	1
1.4	40	2
2.1	60	3
2.8	80	4
3.5	100	5
4.2	120	6
4.9	140	7
5.6	160	8
6.3	180	9
7.0	200	10

Table 2.3. Amount of sugar necessary to create a specific amount of alcohol for 1 gallon or 4 liters

White/Brown sugar (oz.)	White/Brown sugar (g)	Alcohol obtained (%)
2.7	76	1
5.3	150	2
8	227	3
10.7	303	4
13	368	5
16	454	6
18.7	530	7
21.3	604	8
24	680	9
26	737	10

Table 2.3 shows the amount of sugar necessary to generate a given ABV in 1 gallon (4 L) of liquid.

Alternative Sources of Sugar

You can experiment with various sugar sources, such as maple syrup, honey, molasses, commercial fruit syrups, malt extract syrup, and others, for a variety of flavors. When using these sugar sources, I follow a simple generic rule. It's quite workable due to the variations in these ingredients' production, water content, types of sugars present, and so on.

The rule is:

> 1 pound (455 g) honey, maple and other syrups, molasses, and similar sugar sources per 1 gallon (4 L) = around 5% (ABV)

Note that molasses is only about 70 percent fermentable sugars, and this number can go as low as 40 percent for blackstrap molasses. I would use 1¼ pounds (567 g) of molasses per gallon to get 5 to 6 percent ABV. I don't use blackstrap molasses for fermentation.

I hope I kept things simple.

On the Use of Wild Yeast

If you intend to make vinegar from homemade alcoholic ferments such as berry or fruit wines, herbal meads, or wild beers, then we need to talk a bit about wild yeast. Since this book is about vinegars, I've tried to keep this section brief. There is a whole chapter dedicated to wild yeast–harvesting in *The Wildcrafting Brewer*.

Most people who are into making beers, wines, and other alcoholic beverages purchase their yeast online or at their local brewing supply store. Commercial yeasts imbue specific flavors and also allow you to determine the percentage of alcohol you can expect after a full fermentation. As a wildcrafter, I see wild yeast and their associated flavors as a beautiful representation of my local terroir (flavors from the land).

Some people will tell you that wild yeast will ferment up to a point and then die (usually after they've generated around 5 to 6 percent alcohol), but that hasn't been my experience. I've had some wild ferments reach well over 10 percent alcohol—such is the case when I use yeast from my local elderberries. Besides, an alcoholic content of 5 to 6 percent is perfect for making vinegar.

As you'll see in the following pages, I like to use yeast starters to kick off an alcoholic fermentation. The idea is to introduce a large amount of yeast before any bacteria that could spoil the ferment has time to multiply. By doing so, you really increase your chances for a successful fermentation.

You don't always need a starter, such as when you make vinegar from apple scraps (Method 2: Raw Fermentation: Apple Scraps Vinegar). Sometimes, I just let the wild yeast in the ingredients do its thing. A yeast starter is useful when you are not sure how much yeast your ingredients have or when you have to boil your ingredients to extract flavors, thus killing any existing yeast.

Wild yeast is not difficult to collect. Yeast spores are present everywhere—in the air we breathe, in the soil, and on flowers, berries, fruits, and specific plants. As I continue to experiment with brewing, I keep discovering more and more sources of wild yeasts. For example, I recently gave a webinar about making herbal brews. For educational purposes, I made 10 different wild yeast starters using dandelion flowers, blueberries, pine needles, juniper berries (*Juniperus californica*), and so on. Every single one had a successful fermentation.

The key to foraging wild yeast is to find it in high enough quantity to make a good starter. I remember reading a book that recommended harvesting wild yeast by placing the liquid outside to ferment, in hopes that yeast spores in the air would somehow decide to make a home in it. But I didn't experience any success with that method. After a few days, I would see mold form on the surface of the solution, and the smell became unpleasant enough that I did not want to risk drinking any of it.

To keep the harvesting of wild yeast simple, I recommend that you stick with fruits and berries. You can collect them in nature or purchase them at the store. Yeast is attracted by sugar, so you'll have a much better chance of harvesting sufficient quantities of wild yeast from sweet fruits such as pineapple, apples, pears, and the like.

I'll give you another tip. You've probably noticed that some fruits and berries like grapes, blueberries, prickly pears, plums, and similar have a whitish bloom on their skin. This bloom is partly natural wax, but it also contains a lot of yeasts. My local elderberries and juniper berries have a substantial amount of this white bloom, which helps a lot in making good starters.

To help you on your fermentation journey, here are some good sources of wild yeasts:

> Plums, grapes, and other fruits that have a white bloom. You can get them from your garden or farmers market. Make sure they're organic.
> Apple, pears, and lemons. You don't want wax on the skin, so inspect them and choose organic, too. I've never tried oranges or grapefruits.

Pineapple. The yeast is mostly present on the skin.

Gingerroot. Must be organic. Some of the ginger I find locally in stores doesn't work for fermentation. I suspect the food is irradiated to kill potential microorganisms and insects.

Juniper berries.

Elderberries.

Wild grapes.

Elderflowers.

Blueberries.

Blackberries.

Figs.

Prickly pear fruits.

Raw honey. Though a good source of wild yeast, you'll need true raw honey from someone who has a beehive. Most "raw" honey sold commercially, even at farmers markets, is pasteurized at low temperatures.

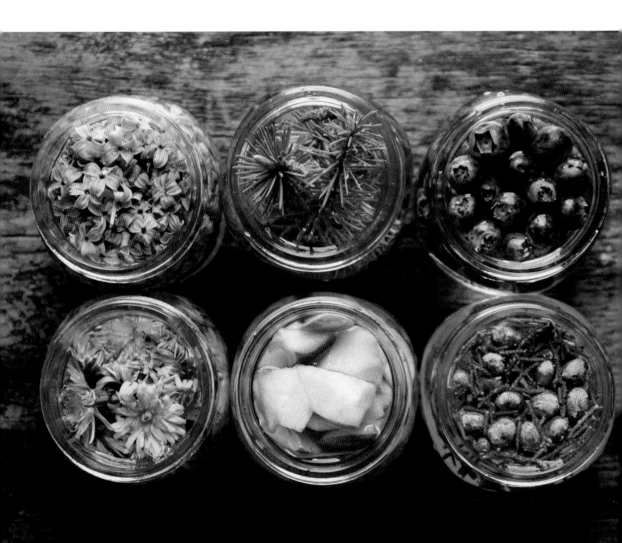

MAKING A WILD YEAST STARTER

The idea behind making a yeast starter is to create a solution that dramatically increases the amount of yeast by feeding it with sugar before "pitching it" (placing it) into your brew. The large quantity of yeast pretty much ensures a successful fermentation.

The method I presently use is almost 100 percent effective. You can substitute the gingerroot with whole blueberries or grapes, pineapple scraps, juniper berries, plum skin, and so on (see the list of possible sources in "On the Use of Wild Yeast," page 55). Note that some yeast sources, such as ginger or juniper berries, may add flavors to your brew. This is generally not an excessive effect. You can even create yeast starter mixes with the intention of accentuating certain flavors or adding character.

Procedure

1. Make a sweet solution composed of around 15 percent sugar and 85 percent water by volume. You can use less than 15 percent sugar—the basic rule is that you want the liquid to taste quite sweet. I like to use store-bought, filtered water because tap water may contain chlorine. Honey or maple syrup can be used, too. If I use a ½-pint jar (240 ml) to create a starter, I'll typically use ¾ cup (180 ml) water and around 0.8 ounces (23 g) white sugar.

2. Pour the solution into a clean bottle or jar. Pasteurizing the container before use by placing it in boiling water for 10 minutes or more is a good practice and will increase your chances of success, but from my experience it's not a must. Washing the bottle or jar with soap and water works well, too.

3. Peel the gingerroot (or otherwise prepare foraged yeast sources) and place the skins in the container with the sugar-water solution.

4. You don't want flies or undesirable bacteria to contaminate your starter, but you need to let fermentation gases escape. If you use a bottle, it is a good idea to use an airlock. For jars, you can use a regular lid and band, just don't screw it too tightly.

5. Shake the container 2 or 3 times a day. If you used a jar, screw the lid on tight before shaking, then unscrew a bit. Around 3 to 5 days later (less in hot weather) you will notice some bubbling in the solution. Congratulations, your fermentation is active!

6. Add some of the wild yeast starter into the liquid you want to ferment. I use around ½ to ¾ cup (120 to 180 ml) of starter for 1 gallon (4 L) of brew. Some recipes I've seen online use 1 cup (240 ml) per gallon (4 L). The consensus seems to be between ½ to 1 cup (120 to 240 ml).

Yeast starters (*clockwise from upper-left*): lilac flower, pine tips, blueberries, juniper berries, apple scraps, dandelion flowers.

I'm so used to making wild yeast starters that these days I just screw the band and lid quite tightly then burp and shake the contents as necessary. A couple of times daily is usually the norm.

If you don't use your starter right away, you can store it in the fridge for a week or two. The low temperature will slow down the fermentation process. Starters are so easy to make that I don't store them for long. I prefer to make new ones.

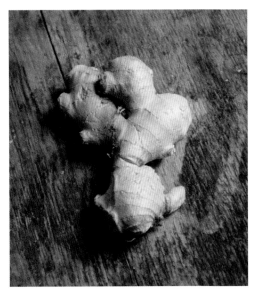

Organic gingerroot.

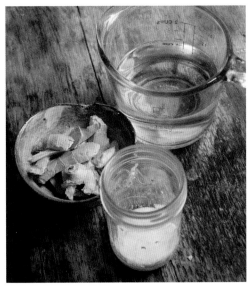

Yeast starter ingredients: 20% sugar (or honey), 80% water (not tap water), and gingerroot skins (that's where the yeast is).

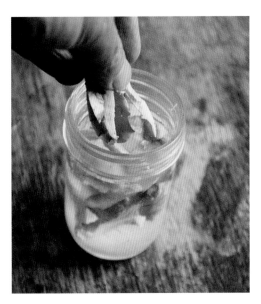

Combine the ingredients in a jar.

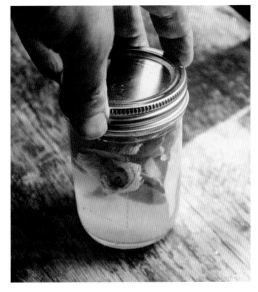

Close the lid, but not too tightly. Shake 3 to 4 times a day.

Making Vinegar from Store-Bought Organic Juice

Let's practice! Turning store-bought organic juices into vinegars is a neat way to explore flavors and start experimenting. You can find all kinds of pasteurized juices, such as apple, cranberry, blackberry, currant, pomegranate, and various blends. The method detailed here will apply to any pasteurized store-bought juice.

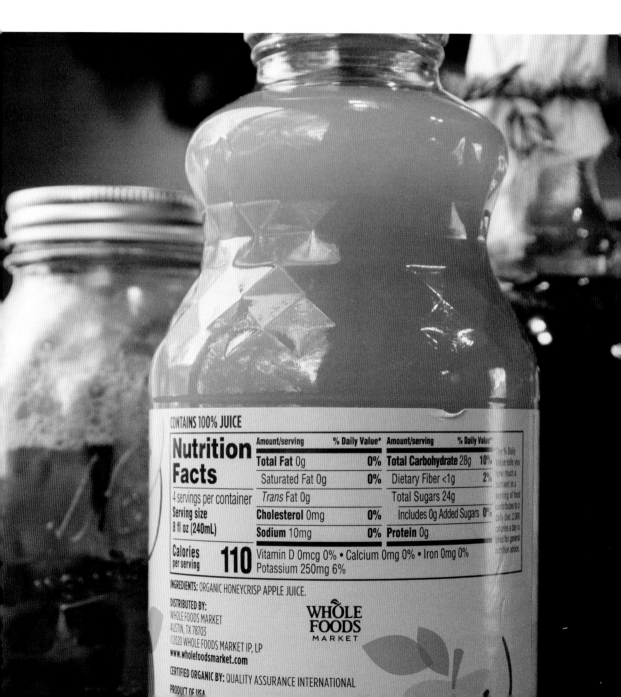

Make sure to read the label when you purchase your juice. I've learned so much about the low standards of our modern food industry while examining juice labels. Check if the juice was made from concentrate and whether the ingredients include corn syrup, artificial flavors or colors, or additives such as ascorbic acid and citric acid. Ideally, your label should list the ingredients as: organic (something) juice.

Note that it's okay if some sugar is added. If you make vinegar from organic cranberry juice, for example, the amount of natural sugar in the berries is usually not enough to produce the right amount of alcohol. You'll need to add some sugar anyway.

The key to figuring out how to ferment the juice and make vinegar can be found on the nutrition label, which lists how much sugar is in the beverage.

For example, I purchased an organic apple juice whose label indicated that the amount of sugar per serving was 0.85 ounces (24 g). The bottle had four 8-ounce (240-ml) servings. Thus, the total amount of juice in the bottle (4 servings) was 1 quart (1 L) and the total amount of sugar was 3.4 ounces (96 g).

If you look at table 2.2 (page 52), 3.5 ounces (100 g) of sugar per quart (1 L) should give you around 5 percent ABV. This is perfectly fine for making vinegar. But as I've mentioned, I usually aim for around 7 percent ABV in my alcoholic ferments, knowing that I can expect a bit more than 5 percent acidity in my vinegar after the conversion from alcohol to acetic acid (see "Determining Acidity," page 33).

Continuing this example with organic apple juice, in order to achieve 7 percent ABV, which requires 4.9 ounces (135 g) of sugar per quart (1 L), I add 1.5 ounces (43 g) of sugar.

In summary, without all the mathematics:

I went to the store and purchased a 1-quart (1 L) bottle of organic juice that contained 3.4 ounces (96 g) of sugar. This is enough to produce a beverage with 5 percent ABV, but I decided to add more sugar so I could achieve 7 percent ABV and, thereby, a vinegar with a bit over 5 percent acidity. I needed to add 1.5 ounces (43 g) of sugar for a total of 4.9 ounces (135 g) for the quart (1 L).

STORE-BOUGHT JUICE VINEGAR

Here is the basic procedure for making vinegar from a store-bought juice once you have determined the amount of sugar you need to add.

Procedure

Transfer your organic juice, sugar added as necessary, into an appropriately sized bottle. You want to make sure you have enough space to add some starter. If necessary, you may need to get rid of (drink!) some of the juice.

For a quart (1 L) of juice, add around 3 tablespoons (45 ml) of an active starter (Making a Wild Yeast Starter). As an alternative, you can simply use commercial wine or champagne yeast. One small packet is usually good for 5 gallons (20 L)—you don't need much. Don't use bread yeast, as it will affect the flavors negatively.

Insert an airlock on the bottle, or place a clean paper towel on top secured by a rubber band. If you use a paper towel, gently shake the contents daily. This is a good way to avoid mold or other spoilage issues in the beginning of the fermentation process, as the surface of the liquid will be in contact with oxygen. It's well worth investing in an airlock, because it really minimizes the risk of spoilage.

Ferment until very little fermentation gases are escaping through the airlock, which is a sign that the alcoholic fermentation is pretty much complete. It takes between 10 and 15 days, depending on the temperature.

To turn the contents into vinegar, transfer it into a regular jar or similar container.

Add around 20 percent by volume of unpasteurized vinegar and a bit of mother if you have it. Place a paper towel or clean towel on top and secure it with a rubber band or string.

Within 2 to 3 weeks, you should have a beautiful amber-orange mother on top. Wait another 3 to 4 weeks, then taste. If you are satisfied, bottle the vinegar and age it for 2 to 3 months or more before using it. Aging will mellow the flavors, but it's not a must. Store the mother if you want to use it to create more vinegar.

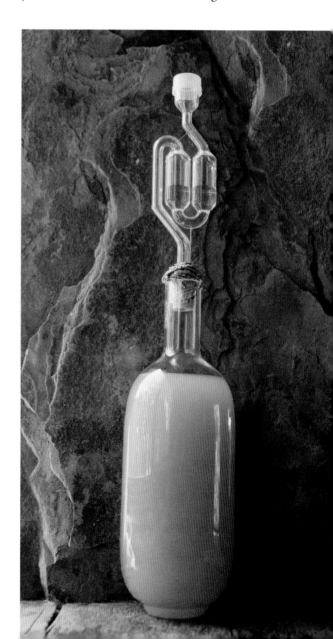

BLACKBERRY WINE VINEGAR

You can make this recipe with foraged or store-bought berries. Personally, I like to use wild berries. I think they have more flavor and I can also forage them when they're at their prime.

This is a good example of making a wine with the sole intent of making vinegar. The "secret" is to keep the amount of alcohol quite low. Between 5 and 9 percent is perfect. To make this kind of vinegar, I usually aim for around 7 to 8 percent alcohol, which will result in a vinegar with 5 or 6 percent acidity.

As we've seen, the amount of sugar used in the wine making process will determine the amount of alcohol obtained. The yeast will "eat" the sugar and convert it to alcohol. As shown in table 2.1 (page 52), blackberries only have enough sugar to make 2 to 3 percent alcohol, which is too low to make vinegar. Thus, you'll need to add enough sugar to get an additional 5 percent potential alcohol.

For 1 quart (1 L) of liquid, you need 0.7 ounces (18 g) of sugar to obtain 1 percent alcohol (see table 2.2, page 53). So 5 percent alcohol will require 3.5 ounces (100 g) of sugar. For this recipe, the wild yeast starter is optional. Blackberries usually have natural yeast on their skin, but I like to use a yeast starter to kick off the fermentation. The faster start guarantees success.

Ingredients for a 1-quart jar (1 L)

30 ounces (850 g) blackberries (will provide around 2¼ cups (530 ml) of juice)

3.5 ounces (100 g) sugar

1½ cups (360 ml) water

2 tablespoons (30 ml) wild yeast starter or wine or champagne yeast (follow manufacturer's direction on amount)

Flavoring herbs such as 3 to 4 mugwort leaves or 1 to 2 dried yarrow flowers (optional)

Procedure

1. Clean the berries briefly in cold water and remove any spoiled or rotting ones.
2. Place the berries into a large bowl and crush with your hands to extract the juice (you can also use a blender). If you crush the berries by hand, it may take around 15 minutes to do a good job. It's a good idea to wear gloves so you don't end up with reddish-purple hands.
3. Add the water and sugar to the crushed berries.
4. Strain the mash. I like to use flour sack kitchen towels, but you can use whatever works. The resulting liquid should fill most of a quart (1 L) bottle.
5. Add the wild yeast starter and a bit of dried mugwort and yarrow if desired. Remove the flavoring herbs after 4 or 5 days.
6. Cover the bottle with a clean towel or paper towel and leave the contents to ferment. Stir or shake it

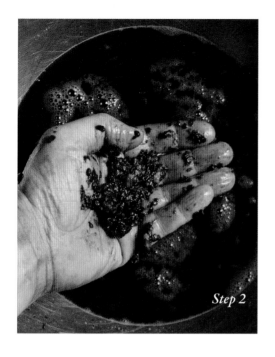

Step 2

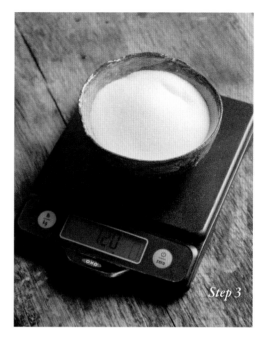

Step 3

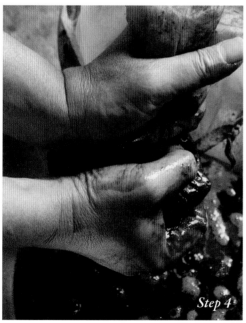

Step 4

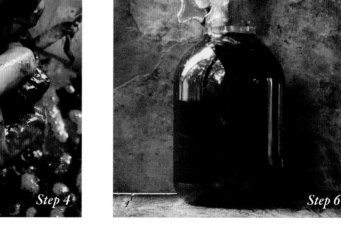

Step 6

slightly each day for the first 2 weeks, then let the wine turn to vinegar naturally over the next 6 to 8 weeks. For a better chance of success or to speed up the process, you can add a bit of mother and some unpasteurized vinegar (20 percent by volume or more).

Herbal Mead Vinegar

These types of honey-based beverages are perfect for exploring local flavors or even creating concoctions that represent whole environments, such as the mountains, your local forest, or, heck, even your backyard. You can use honey or maple syrup; either will make a delicious drink.

I made the vinegar described here when I visited my friends Tara and Mark, who run an organic farm in Colorado (Esoterra Culinary Garden) and grow a lot of savory herbs for local restaurants. I decided to make a drink that would feature some of the herbs and flavors of Colorado. It was pretty much a mix of the local wild herbs and the organic herbs they grow on the farm.

To make a delicious drink, the skill is to determine the right quantity of each plant so the final blend is delightful. It may take some experimentation in the beginning, but over time you'll be able to create drinkable masterpieces.

For example, too much yarrow would make it too bitter. In this case, the various mints I collected made up around 70 percent of the blend and the other herbs were just there as savory accents. You can chop or bruise the herbs, which helps with flavor extraction.

I used the following herbs:

Wild yarrow
3 types of wild mints
(one was similar to peppermint and another seemed to be a cross of peppermint and water mint [*Mentha aquatic*])

Regular and wild fennel
(*Foeniculum vulgare*)
Wild rose hips
Oregano (just a touch)
Fresh cilantro
Sage flowers
Organic lemons (3 sliced lemons for a gallon [4 L])

To calculate the amount of sugar, I used my super simplistic "Neanderthal" rule, which is: 1 pound (455 g) of honey or maple syrup per gallon (4 L) of liquid. That amount yields around 5 percent alcohol. The wild yeast was already present on many of the ingredients (yarrow, mints, and lemons). Pure raw honey purchased from someone who has beehives will also contain wild yeast. Most store-bought raw honeys are pasteurized at a low temperature, and so they will not contain wild yeast.

To make this mead vinegar, I use a bit more than 1¼ pounds (567 g) of honey per gallon (4 L). This ratio yields a mead with around 7 percent alcohol which, once turned into vinegar, gives me 5.5 percent acidity.

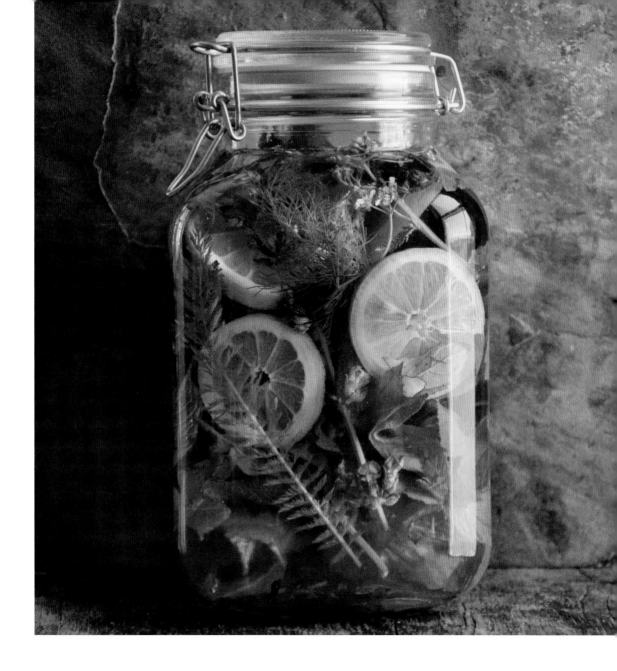

You can use a container with an airlock, but in this case I like to use a jar with a clamp-top lid. The main alcohol fermentation period lasts around 3 weeks. I strain the herbs out after 2 to 3 days, and I shake, stir, and burp the contents twice a day for the first 10 days.

Once the alcoholic fermentation has slowed down, I open the jar, secure a clean towel on top, and let the natural *Acetobacter* do their work. The whole process takes around 2 months. For a better chance of success or to speed up the process, you can add a bit of mother and some unpasteurized vinegar (20 percent by volume or more).

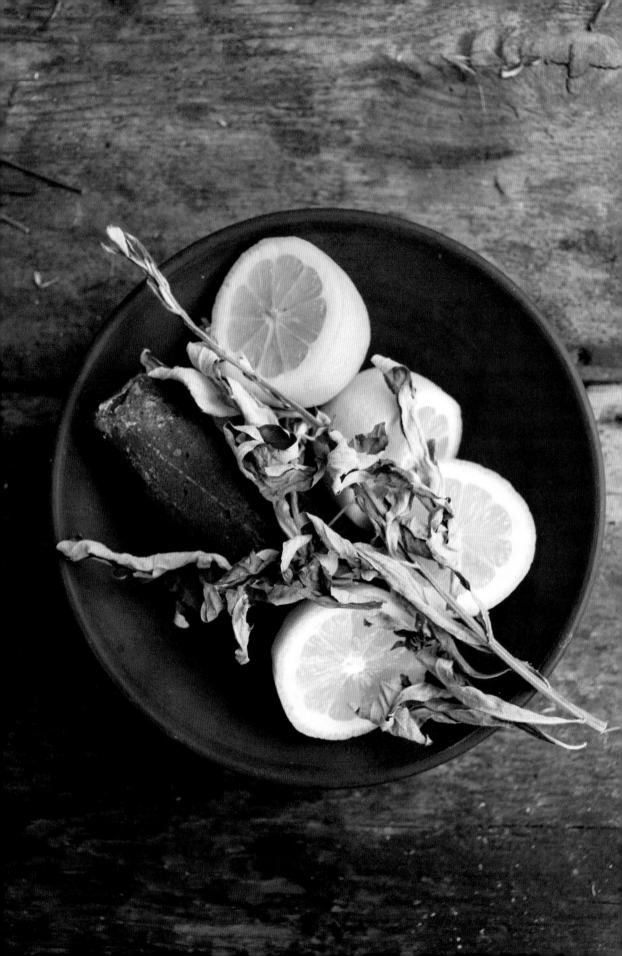

MUGWORT BEER VINEGAR

Mugwort beer is one of the classics in my book *The Wildcrafting Brewer*, and it's the first wild beer I turned into vinegar. Historically, before the appearance of hops, mugwort was one of the main bittering and aromatic herbs used by Celts and Vikings to flavor beer. I would not be surprised if they used vinegars similar to this one to pickle food.

To this day, I make sure I always have some of this vinegar in stock in my pantry. It's similar to an excellent apple cider vinegar but with a slight bitterness and hints of lemon and sage. If you are interested in exploring the world of wild brews and their culinary possibilities, I have lots of step-by-step tutorials with photos in *The Wildcrafting Brewer*.

The sugar used in this recipe should yield around 7 percent ABV.

Ingredients for a ½-gallon and a 1-quart jar (2 L, 1 L)

½ gallon (2 L) water (not tap), more if needed
0.15 ounce (4.5 g) dried mugwort
Juice from 2 lemons
10 ounces (280 g) brown sugar
⅓ cup (80 ml) wild yeast starter
  (Making a Wild Yeast Starter) or beer yeast
  (follow manufacturer's directions)

Procedure

1. Boil the water, mugwort, lemon juice, and brown sugar for 30 minutes in a covered pot, then place the pot in cold water and cool the solution until it is lukewarm.
2. Add the yeast, stir briefly, then strain the liquid into a ½-gallon (2 L) bottle. It's okay if you need to add a bit more water to compensate for evaporation, but fill it to the bottle's neck.
3. Place an airlock on top of the bottle and ferment until you get very little to no gases escaping through the airlock. This is a sign

that the alcoholic fermentation is pretty much complete. It takes around 2 weeks.

4. To turn the brew into vinegar, transfer the contents into a large jar or similar container. I use a ½-gallon (2-L) jar and 1-quart (1-L) jar for this recipe, and each jar ended up nearly two thirds full.
5. It's completely optional but for a better chance of success or to speed up the process, add around 20 percent by volume of unpasteurized vinegar to your jars, and some vinegar mother if you have it.
6. Place a paper towel or clean towel on top of each container and secure it with a rubber band or string.
7. Within 2 to 3 weeks, you should have a beautiful amber-orange mother on top. Wait another 3 to 4 weeks, taste, and bottle if you're satisfied. Age the vinegar for 2 to 3 months or more before using it. Aging will mellow the flavors, but it's not a must. Store the mother if you want to use it to create more vinegar.

ELDERBERRY WINE VINEGAR

This is the recipe I use to make a traditional elderberry wine. In this case, we'll turn it into vinegar. I employ the European method, which uses raw (not boiled) fermentation. (You can learn more about this method in my book *The Wildcrafting Brewer.*) The final product will hover around 14 percent ABV and will need to be diluted with water by 50 percent to make the vinegar.

Ingredients for a ½-gallon jug (2 L)

1½ pounds (680 g) elderberries

1 pound (455 g) granulated white sugar

6 cups (1.4 L) spring water or distilled water

½ teaspoon (2.5 ml) citric acid or juice of 1 lemon

1½ cups (360 ml) unpasteurized vinegar (or you can use store-bought raw apple cider vinegar)

Procedure

1. With clean hands, remove the berries from the stems and crush them in a bowl. Let the mash rest for 30 minutes or so, then strain the juice though a cheesecloth or sieve.
2. In a clean bowl, combine the juice, sugar, water, and citric acid. No need to add yeast; it's already present in the juice from the elderberry skins.
3. Place the liquid in a ½-gallon (2 L) bottle fitted with an airlock and let it ferment for 3 months.
4. Dilute the fermented wine with water. I use a ratio of 50 percent wine and 50 percent water.

5. Transfer the diluted wine into a glass container, then add the unpasteurized vinegar.
6. Cover the container with a clean towel and place it in a somewhat shady place. Within 3 to 4 weeks, it should have a beautiful mother floating on top. Wait another couple of weeks, then strain and bottle the contents. Store the mother if you want to use it to create more vinegar. Age the vinegar for 2 to 3 months or more before using it. Aging will mellow the flavors, but it's not a must.

You can be a purist and, because this is a raw fermentation, decide not to add the unpasteurized vinegar (or store-bought raw apple cider vinegar). That way, you will end up with 100-percent elderberry wine vinegar. After transferring the diluted wine into a jar covered with a clean towel, the *Acetobacter* already present in the wine should naturally turn the contents into vinegar in about 6 to 8 weeks. I've never tried this method, but in theory, it should work.

Another possibility for making this vinegar is to cut the amount of sugar in the recipe by half. This should yield a wine with around 7 percent ABV, which will not need to be diluted. Follow the same procedure for the alcoholic fermentation, but cut the fermentation time to 1½ months. When that's finished, transfer the wine into a jar and cover it with a clean towel, and then continue with the remainder of the vinegar-making process.

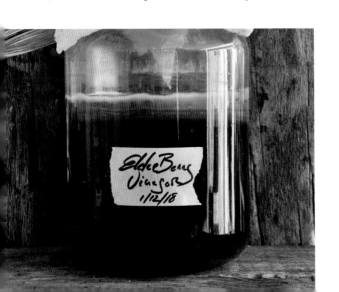

TURNING A MASH INTO VINEGAR: PLUMS

Some fruits or berries, such as plums, peaches, pawpaws, and manzanita berries, cannot be juiced easily. One way around this problem is to make a mash. A mash can be made using a regular food processor. Just make sure to remove the seeds or pits first.

The same principles as other alcoholic ferments destined to become vinegar hold true here: You'll need 3 to 9 percent alcohol (7 percent is ideal in order to end up with a 5 percent acidity vinegar). Based on table 2.1 (page 52), fermented plums can reach 6–8 percent ABV. I'm sure that's true if you pick them from a garden tree when they are fully ripe, but store-bought plums are not always very sweet. For this project, I estimated a possible 5 percent ABV ferment from my purchased plums. Even if you use store-bought ingredients, you can still impart true local (wild) flavors with additional ingredients, like I did in this recipe with mugwort and juniper berries.

You need to add some water, too; otherwise, you'll end up fermenting a thick paste that will be difficult to strain into a liquid vinegar. In this case I added 25 percent water, but by doing so, I also diluted the amount of sugar in the mash and needed to add more.

Here are the calculations I made to create my vinegar: 75 percent of my mash is from plums, which I estimated could reach 5 percent ABV. By adding that 25 percent water without sugar, my mash would now reach around 3.75 percent ABV, which is not enough. Thus, I needed to add enough sugar to add another 3.5 percent potential ABV to the mash so the final ferment would be a tad more than 7 percent ABV. And there's no need to add yeast—wild yeast is already present on the plums and berries.

Ingredients for a ¾-gallon jar (3 L)

7½ cups (1.8 L) plum mash
   (estimated 5 percent potential ABV)
2½ cups (600 ml) water
5.9 ounces (168 g) added sugar
7 mugwort leaves for flavoring
10 to 15 California juniper berries
   (unripe and crushed) for flavoring
2½ cups (600 ml) unpasteurized vinegar

Procedure

Once you've created the mash, combine with the water, sugar, mugwort, and juniper berries and ferment the mash for a bit more than 2 weeks in a large jar. Briefly open the jar and stir the contents a couple of times daily. When the fermentation is complete, strain the mash using a flour sack kitchen towel or another fine material.

Transfer the liquid into the appropriate-sized jar and add around 20 percent unpasteurized vinegar and a bit of mother if you have it. Secure a clean towel or paper towel on top. Within 3 to 4 weeks, you should have vinegar with a beautiful mother floating on top. Wait another couple of weeks, then strain and bottle the contents. Age the vinegar for 2 to 3 months or more before using it. Aging will mellow the flavors, but it's not a must.

As an alternative, you can skip adding a starter (unpasteurized vinegar) and let the *Acetobacter* already present slowly turn the mash into vinegar. I have used both methods and they each worked very well. It takes a bit longer without a culture starter.

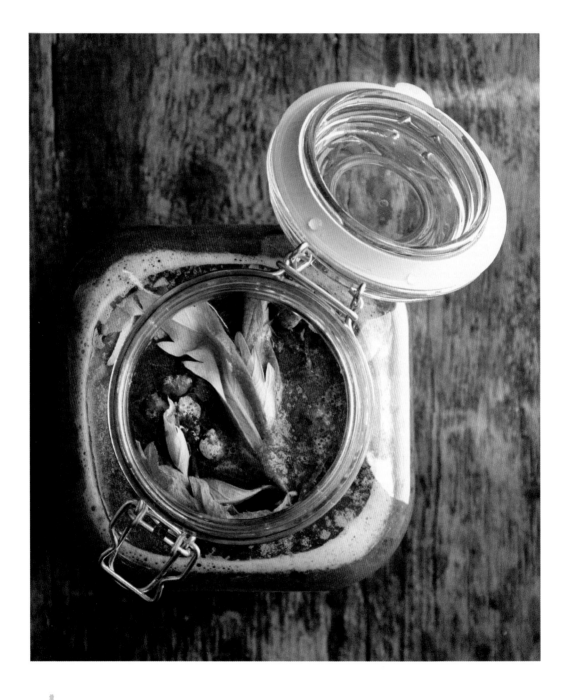

WITCH'S BREW VINEGAR

A couple of months ago, I made a sort of medicinal shamanic brew for one of my wild beer workshops. As I was working on this book at the time, I thought it would be kind of interesting to turn it into a vinegar. I mean, it's kind of cool. . . . Where can you purchase some witch's brew vinegar?

I used turkey tail mushrooms (*Trametes versicolor*), which are said to boost the immune system. Mushroom tea is basically my base liquid for the brew. You'll also find willow bark, used in the old days to reduce fever. Willow bark contains the same compound as aspirin (salicin) and was used in the Middle Ages as a bittering agent for beers. Then, following my inner wizard, I added some mugwort—which is a traditional ingredient in wild beers and said to induce vivid or lucid dreaming—and some horehound (*Marrubium vulgare*), which helps the respiratory system.

The amount of sugar used in this recipe should yield around 7.5 percent ABV. The procedure is somewhat similar to the Mugwort Beer Vinegar procedure.

Ingredients for a 1-gallon bottle (4 L)

1.2 ounces (34 g) turkey tail mushrooms

1½ gallons (6 L) water (not tap)

0.25 ounce (7 g) dried mugwort

0.05 ounces (1.5 g) horehound

0.1 ounces (3 g) willow bark

2 spider legs (not really, but it sounds great and witchy)

3 lemons, juiced

1¼ pounds (567 g) brown sugar

Beer yeast (follow manufacturer's instructions) or ½ cup (120 ml) of wild yeast starter (Making a Wild Yeast Starter)

1 quart (1 L) unpasteurized vinegar

Procedure

1. Place your turkey tail mushrooms into a pot with the water, cover the pot, and bring the water to a boil. Reduce the heat and simmer very slowly for a couple of hours. Simmer until you have about 1 gallon (4 L) of liquid.

2. Add the mugwort, horehound, willow bark, lemon juice, and brown sugar and continue to simmer for 30 minutes in the covered pot. When done, place the pot in cold water and cool the solution to lukewarm. Add the yeast, then strain into a 1-gallon (4 L) bottle.

3. Place an airlock on top of the bottle and ferment until very little to no fermentation gases escape through the airlock, which is a sign that the alcoholic fermentation is pretty much complete. It takes around 2 weeks.

4. To turn the brew into vinegar, transfer the contents to a large jar or similar container. In this case, I used a gallon (4 L) jar and 1-quart (1 L) jar. Each jar ended up just over three-quarters full.

5. To each jar, add around 20 percent by volume of unpasteurized vinegar and some vinegar mother if you have it.

6. Place a paper towel or clean towel on top of each jar and secure with a rubber band or string.
7. Within 2 to 3 weeks, you should have a beautiful amber mother on top. Wait another 3 to 4 weeks, then taste. If you're satisfied, bottle the vinegar and age it for 2 to 3 months or more before using it. Aging will mellow the flavors, but it's not a must. Store the mother if you want to use it to create more vinegar.

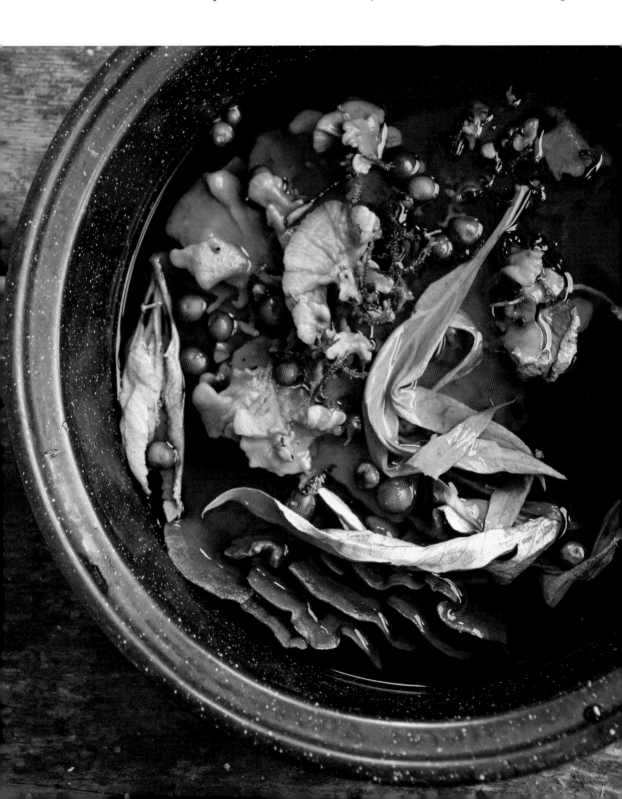

CHAPTER 3

The Quest for Local Flavors:
Infused Vinegars

I'll tell you a little secret. Yes, you now know how to make incredibly tasty vinegars from scratch, but the flavors you can impart through the infusion of spices, savory herbs, fruits, and berries are hard to beat.

As an interesting experiment, last year I made some Elderberry Wine Vinegar as well as apple cider vinegar infused with elderberries. I then had some of my experienced students and forager friends taste them to see if they could identify which was which. Not everyone was able to recognize the elderberry wine vinegar for what it was, but the elderberry-infused vinegar was immediately recognizable and an instant hit.

Don't get me wrong. The wine vinegar was well liked, but some confused it with a regular, high-quality red wine vinegar. On the other hand, the infused vinegar had that very distinct earthy, fruity, and slightly tart taste of elderberries, even though the base vinegar was a regular, good-quality unpasteurized apple cider vinegar.

There is beauty in both. Homemade vinegars made from fermented wines, beers, meads, and spirits are themselves outstanding compared to regular store-bought products. But through infusion, you can really home in on the savory characteristics of the ingredients you use.

That said, by mixing the two methods you can achieve some truly priceless and exquisite results. An elderberry wine vinegar infused with dehydrated elderberries will be far tastier than either on its own, and, in my opinion, a true savory representation of the berries.

One advantage of making infused vinegars is the fun and simplicity of the process. It's also much faster to make, as you don't have to go through the whole process of alcoholic fermentation. You just need to place the base vinegar and your flavoring ingredients into a jar or similar container, cover it, and wait for a few weeks.

Some recipes call for the vinegar to be heated slightly in order to extract the flavors or for food safety. For example, wild mushrooms and elderberries typically should be heated before consumption. But, as you'll see, most of my recipes use a raw process with unpasteurized vinegar and fresh ingredients.

Exploring Your Local Terroir

In terms of experimenting with your environment and researching local flavors, making infused vinegars are even better than making vinegars from scratch. You just need a good base vinegar to start. From there, you can attempt to infuse anything as long as it's not poisonous or unhealthy.

Not all the concoctions you put together will work, but with experience and taking care to learn from your failures, you'll be able to create some incredibly complex and tasty blends. For example, it took me years to figure out my mountain blend, which has up to 12 different ingredients in various proportions.

It's completely possible to make infused vinegars that capture a moment in time and the genuine flavors of a specific place. It's a creative process that is a true meditation. The first stage involves taking several long walks and doing research into the local plants. It's very much about getting a sense of what's growing there and the flavor profiles of those plants.

The second stage is becoming acquainted with the "spirit" of the place. Every place has a spirit—the ecosystem creates its own personality. I think we're all aware of this on some level. If you spend time in nature, you get the feel of a particular place: Some places give you a sense of serenity, awe, or happiness while others may seem depressing, dangerous, or lacking in soul.

It's similar with taste. Once a place inspires you and you've done your research into the edible local flora, empty your mind and let the place talk to you from a flavor perspective.

For example, the local mountains close to where I used to live in Southern California were mostly composed of pinyon pine (*Pinus edulis*) and white fir (*Abies concolor*), but there was also a decent amount of mugwort and yarrow. Then there were flavor accents such as fennel, ponderosa pine (*P. ponderosa*), juniper, various sagebrushes, and sages.

My favorite inspirational location in those mountains speaks to me of wisdom and serenity—there is a sense of old age associated with it.

I try to infuse all of those qualities, flavors, perceptions, and inspiration into the vinegar I create. I usually start with a good-quality apple cider vinegar and infuse it with pinyon pine branches, white fir needle, and crushed unripe juniper berries, which will give the vinegar lemony and tangerine flavors with hints of pine. Mugwort and yarrow are ancestral herbs used in the old continent by Vikings and Celts as brewing ingredients, but they also have medicinal and spiritual properties. I gather mugwort in fall, when the plant has deep, complex flavors that I associate with aging. I also fancy the mature plant as wiser than a young plant, which has a very youthful flavor profile.

My mountain blend varies each year, meaning it is a true representation of place and time. If we had some good rain, I may find elderflowers, manzanita berries, or even mushrooms. A typical blend may contain over 12 different ingredients in various ratios.

True to my perception that the place evokes old age and the wisdom associated with it, I'll age that vinegar much longer than any others—up to a couple of years with all the ingredients.

In the end, your vinegar becomes more than just a vinegar. You will have established a personal spiritual connection and a sense of place. This is how real food should be.

Shelf Life and Storage

One of the main differences between a vinegar made from fermentation and a vinegar infusion is the shelf life. For example, a properly stored elderberry wine vinegar will last years, while one infused with dehydrated elderberries should be consumed within a year for optimum flavor.

The consensus seems to be that most infused vinegars will retain optimal flavor for 5 to 6 months or up to a year with good storage, but of course you will have some exceptions. Pine, fir, and spruce products tend to keep their savory qualities for a long time. For example, I usually infuse my Mountains Vinegar for 6 months to a year, then strain it and age it for another 6 months before consuming. I get the best flavors that way.

The reason most infused vinegars don't keep as long as regular vinegars is because the flavors of the infusion come from organic compounds which, unlike the vinegar itself, tend to deteriorate over time. I once made an infused wild mint vinegar that tasted like a regular apple cider vinegar a year later. Well, sort of. . . . It still had a tiny bit of flavor, but it was nothing compared to the freshly infused vinegar.

The best way to preserve flavor over time is proper storage. When you bottle your infused vinegar, fill the bottle as much as possible to avoid excessive exposure to air, and make sure it is tightly sealed.

Store in a cool, dark place: 65°F (18°C) or below if possible, or in the fridge. If you see any sign of spoilage such as mold, sliminess, or unusual cloudiness, just toss the product. On the good side, this has never happened to me in the 20 years I've been making infused vinegars.

Vinegars for Infusing

You can use any vinegar you like to create an infusion, but it is best to pair specific types of vinegar with the appropriate savory ingredients. For example, a distilled white vinegar infused with elderberries would not work as well as a red wine vinegar or an elderberry wine vinegar. In fact, I never use distilled white vinegar to make infused vinegar. Another bad pairing is balsamic vinegar infused with mint—the two flavors just don't work well. However, a good-quality apple cider vinegar infused with white fir or pinyon pine is heavenly.

The Colorado State University Extension recommends the following vinegars for infusion:

Distilled white vinegar   Champagne vinegar
Apple cider vinegar   Red wine vinegar
White wine vinegar   Balsamic vinegar*

But of course, if you make your own vinegar, your choices are pretty much infinite. Apple cider vinegar works well with fruits and berries, while white wine vinegar or champagne vinegar is usually paired with herbs. However, I often use apple cider vinegar or mead vinegar for herbs and chilies, too. Red wine vinegar can be awesome with strongly flavored ingredients such as black walnuts (*Juglans nigra*), olives, garlic, elderberries, and the like. Rice vinegar is milder and works well with subtle savory ingredients such as seaweeds or mushrooms. From my perspective, there are no real rules.

My only advice with regard to infused vinegars is to use vinegars with at least 5 percent acidity to start with. Some ingredients used to flavor vinegars could reduce the acidity level, and you don't want to end up with a final flavored vinegar that isn't acidic enough and is prone to spoiling.

Flavoring Ingredients

Some of the most common wild (or not) ingredients used for flavoring are:

Fruits and berries (wild or store-bought). Elderberries, sumac berries, manzanita berries, juniper berries, blueberries, blackberries, raspberries, orange, grapefruit, lime or lemon peel.

---

* D. Grubb, E. Shackleton, and M. Bunning, "Making Flavored Vinegar—9.340," Colorado State University Extension, January 2021, https://extension.colostate .edu/topic-areas/nutrition-food-safety-health/flavored-vinegars-and-oils-9-340/.

Fresh herbs. Wild herbs such as mint, fennel, tarragon (*Artemisia dracunculus*), burr chervil (*Anthriscus caucalis*), sweet white clover (*Melilotus albus*). Store-bought herbs such as lemongrass, thyme, parsley (*Petroselinum crispum*), dill, basil, rosemary.

Dried herbs. Bay leaves (I use California bay leaves [*Umbellularia californica*]), mugwort, yarrow, wild sages, and sagebrush (I use California sagebrush [*Artemisia californica*]). A lot of herbs can be used fresh or dried (thyme, rosemary, and the like).

Spices. Peppercorn, black mustard, chilies, cinnamon, vanilla beans.

Seeds. Wild fennel and celery seeds, black mustard seeds, cumin, coriander, dill, fenugreek.

Vegetables. Garlic, fresh peppers (jalapeños, Thai, habaneros, and others), wild or store-bought onions, shallots.

Roots. Ginger, wild mustard (*Sinapis arvensis*), licorice (*Glycyrrhiza glabra*), wild celery (*Apium graveolens*), sassafras (*Sassafras albium*), turmeric (*Curcuma longa*).

Unusual Wildcrafted Ingredients

In my quest for true local flavors, I've successfully used quite a few unusual ingredients to infuse flavors in my vinegars and even create vinegars that are representations of whole environments, such as my California mountains or forest vinegars. You might not find all of these in your immediate area, but they may give you some ideas about what to look for.

Barks. I use roasted oak bark to imbue smoky flavors in some of my lacto-ferments, such as hot sauces, and, of course, in my vinegars. It can make your vinegar taste like it has been aged in a toasted oak barrel. Using roasted oak bark is a good alternative to purchasing an oak barrel if you don't want to spend the money on one. The bark I collect is recycled from fallen oak trees or branches. I'm sure there are other types of bark that could be used—you just need to research it. So far, I've used bark from white oak (*Quercus alba*)and coast live oak (*Q. agrifolia*).

Stems and twigs. I use quite a few sages and other aromatic herbs to create various spice blends or for brewing. Originally, I only used the leaves, but over time I realized that the stems or branches and/or twigs were also highly savory and, instead of wasting the resources, I started to use them for flavoring, as well. The stems, branches, or twigs I've used so far are:

Mugwort stems
California sagebrush stems

Black sage stems
Wild tarragon (*Artemisia dracunculus*) stems
California bay twigs
Sweet white clover stems
White sage (*Salvia apiana*) stems
Epazote (*Dysphania ambrosioides*) stems
Water mint stems
Pinyon pine branches

Pinyon pine is a very interesting flavoring ingredient. You can use the unripe green pine cones or the needles, although the needles have a bitter edge. But what is spectacular are the small branches. You need to remove the needles and split the branches in two lengthwise portions, then place them into the vinegar. The flavor of this vinegar (Pinyon Pine–Infused Vinegar) reminds me of fruity pine candies I used to eat in Belgium as a kid.

Wood. Traditionally, oak has been the wood of choice to flavor vinegar or wine, but there are many other woods that can impart pleasing accents. You don't always need to forage them. You can purchase various wood chips that are normally used for grilling or barbecuing—mesquite, birch, apple, apricot, hickory, and many others—online or in stores. Locally, I forage wood chips from mesquite, figs, oak, and juniper to infuse my wild beers, wines, and vinegars.

Rather than using large pieces of wood, woods chips are much better for infusing flavors. Toast them lightly with a kitchen torch (or your oven) and you'll end up with some interesting smoky accents.

Unripe berries. Some unripe berries have a different flavor profile than the ripe berries. Our California juniper berries are much tastier when green and unripe—they're lemony with strong hints of pine. And unripe, green manzanita berries can be used as a lemon substitute.

Pine, fir, and spruce needles. I use juniper berries to infuse pine flavors, and I use pine or fir needles to infuse lemony or tangerine flavors. All true pine can be used for culinary purposes. Online, you'll find references to ponderosa pine being poisonous, along with trees and conifers that are not from the pine (*Pinus*) family. From my research, this conclusion came from a study related to abortive issues in cattle that ate large quantities of it. Guess what—we're not cattle and we don't eat pounds of it. Ponderosa pine needle tea has been and still is used as a good source of vitamin C. But if you are pregnant, I would not recommend ingesting pine via teas or infused products.

Some evergreens or conifers are not actually pines and should be avoided. These include Norfolk Island pine (*Araucaria heterophylla*) and yew (*Podocarpus macrophyllus*), which is deadly.

Note that not all pine needles will taste lemony. Some can be quite bitter (such as pinyon pine) and others are just tasteless.

Seaweed. If you want your vinegars to taste a tad like the sea, seaweed is wonderful. It's so good that I made a trip to Northern California just to forage some. So far, the seaweeds I've used include wakame (*Undaria pinnatifida*), giant kelp (*Macrocystis pyrifera*), and Mendocino Coast kombu (*Laminaria dentigera*). One of my favorite infused vinegars is made with smoked seaweed. It's absolutely delicious.

Mushrooms. I still have a lot of experimentations to do, but infusing mushrooms to flavor vinegar is definitely worth it in terms of results. Some mushrooms, such as Southern California's local candy caps (*Lactarius rubidus*), can be very aromatic.

Ratio of Ingredients to Vinegar

There are limits as to how much of an ingredient you can infuse in your vinegar. Sometimes it's a matter of taste. For example, an excessive amount of thyme or bay leaves infused in your vinegar is not going to taste great. But the limits can be related to food safety, too. If an ingredient is not acidic enough and you use too much of the herb, it could raise the pH and make your vinegar prone to spoiling.

The National Center for Home Food Preservation guidelines are as follows:

Fresh herbs: 2 to 3 sprigs per pint (2 cups)
Dried herbs: 1 teaspoon (around 9 g) per pint (2 cups)
Fruits: 1 to 2 cups per pint, or 1 orange or lemon peel per pint
Vegetables: 1 to 2 cups per pint
Spices: ½ teaspoon (1.5 g) per pint*

Note for those using the metric system: A cup has a volume of 240 ml, so 2 cups equals a volume of 480 ml, or around 0.5 liter.

For berries (wild or commercial), I use the fruit guideline: 1 to 2 cups per pint (240 to 480 ml).

---

* Elizabeth Andress and Judy Harrison, "Preserving Food: Flavored Vinegars," National Center for Home Food Preservation, June 2011, https://nchfp.uga.edu /publications/uga/uga_flavored_vinegars.pdf.

The guidelines are helpful when we talk about generic ingredients, but I like to go further and calculate the pH of some of the wild ingredients I use. For example, pine, spruce, and fir needles are quite acidic (low pH), and you can therefore use a greater amount. I have no problem using a ratio of 1 part pine or fir needles to 2 parts vinegar. The same would apply to juniper berries. Flavor-wise, I use a greater quantity of dried foraged herbs if the flavors are milder than commercial savory herbs. For example, chickweed has less intense flavors than rosemary. On the contrary, some of the sages or sagebrushes I collect in Southern California have such a pungency that I use much less than the guidelines recommend.

The National Center for Home Food Preservation guidelines are for *infused* vinegars. In chapter 4, you'll find recipes for herb pastes where the ratio of fresh herbs to vinegar is much higher. There are a lot of wild ingredients that are not listed in their guidelines, such as roots, barks, stems, mushrooms, and so on. All the recipes in this book that use ingredients not listed in their guidelines have been pH-tested over time by me.

You can use spices or herb powders, but realize they will probably make your final vinegar quite cloudy.

Infusion Methods

The two main infusion methods are the hot method (heated vinegar) and the cold method (room temperature or refrigerated vinegar). There is another method, the solar method, whereby you place the jar or container of infusing vinegar in the sunshine. The solar heat helps extract the flavors over time. Having lived mostly in Southern California underneath its unforgiving sun, I have never used the solar method because the heat inside the jar would become excessive.

Hot Method

Heat can help extract the flavors from the ingredients you are attempting to infuse. This is especially effective with spices or dried herbs. It's the method I use to make my spicy vinegar with dried chili pods or vinegars with dehydrated elderberries.

This method is fairly easy. Start by heating the vinegar to just below boiling. Meanwhile, if necessary, clean the herbs, spices, vegetables, fruits, or other ingredients you plan to use. You can also chop or bruise savory herbs for optimal extraction. I often cut or poke berries with the tip of a knife so they can release their essence.

Place your ingredients in a clean jar or similar container, then add the hot vinegar. Don't overpack (use the guidelines in "Ratio of Ingredients to Vinegar," page 79). If you are using jars, keep ¼ to ½ inch (0.6–1.3 cm) headspace.

Close the lid and store in a cool, dark place, like a basement or fridge. Taste after a couple of weeks to see if you like it. Most infused vinegars need to be aged for at least a month for optimum flavors, but that's not always the case if you use very flavorful ingredients. It's ultimately up to you—you can taste as you go along and stop aging when you want. If the flavors are too strong, you can always add more vinegar.

When I'm happy with the flavors, I strain the vinegar into a bottle. You can add a sprig or two of fresh herbs or berries for a decorative flourish. You want to minimize the oxygen exposure for long-term storage, so just make sure the bottle is filled up as much as possible. Store in a cool, dark place, like a basement or fridge. Shelf life for optimum flavors is around 6 months and up to a year if the temperature is kept below 65°F (18°C). If you store outside of a refrigerator in a high-room-temperature location, such as in Southern California, you're looking at a few weeks.

Cold Method

This is a very traditional method that I use the most because heat can alter the flavors of many ingredients I infuse, such as pine, fir, juniper berries, spruce, and others. Both pasteurized and raw vinegar have worked for me without any problems.

I try to follow a ratio of 1 part flavoring ingredients to 2 parts vinegar by volume. If I know that the berries, fruits, or other ingredients I want to infuse are quite acidic, I may up the ratio to 1 part infusing matter for 1 part vinegar. A good example would be my white fir needle vinegar. In the past, I tested the pH of a paste made from fresh needles and it was very low. Thus, I use a 1:1 ratio for this vinegar.

The method is as follows: Wash your flavoring ingredients in cold water and remove any bad parts. If you don't forage your ingredients, make sure they're fresh and organic. To better extract flavors, herbs can be bruised, fruits can be chopped, and berries can be crushed or pricked with the tip of a knife.

Place your ingredients in a jar or similar container using 1 part infusing matter and 2 parts vinegar. Close the lid and store in a cool, dark place, like a basement or fridge.

Shake the contents gently at least once a day for the first 3 to 4 days, then about once a week after that. Taste as you go along—you can stop the process anytime. I usually age the vinegar for 3 to 4 weeks, then strain and bottle it.

As explained earlier, you want to minimize oxygen exposure. Fill the bottle as much as possible. Store in a cool, dark place, like a basement or fridge. Shelf life will be around 6 months if the temperature is kept below 65°F (18°C), or a few weeks if the temperature is higher. I don't age raw berry or fruit infusions for more than a month for optimum flavors.

A Note on Flavors

Many of the infused vinegars I make pair savory and aromatic herbs or spices with fruits or berries. For example, in one recipe I add some tasty fresh mugwort to my blueberry-infused vinegar. If you create a recipe from scratch, sometimes you'll need to make a decision about which method to use, or even use both methods. A heated vinegar will be much better for spices, whereas a cold method would be better for other ingredients. As such, you could heat the vinegar, add the spices, let it cool, and then add other flavoring such as berries.

Sterilizing Containers

I've never experienced a problem using unsterilized jars or bottles if they are properly cleaned. But if you are uncertain about the hygiene of the location where you make your vinegar, sterilize the containers you plan to use.

My usual technique for sterilization is to use a water bath canner and place the jars in the rack. If you use a regular pot (without a rack), it's a good idea to place a kitchen towel under the jars or bottles so they don't touch the bottom of the pot directly (they can break). Cover them with warm water so there is about one inch of water above them, then bring the water to a boil for 10 minutes if you live at an elevation less than 1,000 feet (300 m). Add 1 additional minute for each additional 1,000 feet (300 m) of elevation. Table 3.1 shows the time to sterilization for a range of altitudes.

Lids should be properly cleaned with hot water and dish soap. You don't have to do anything with canning bands, as they don't touch the food.

Table 3.1. Sterilization at Various Altitudes

Altitude (ft.)	Altitude (m)	Sterilizing time (minutes)
0–1,000	0–300	10
1,001–2,000	301–600	11
2,001–3,000	601–900	12
3,001–4,000	901–1,200	13
4,001–5,000	1,201–1,500	14
5,001–6,000	1,501–1,800	15
6,001–7,000	1,801–2,100	16
7,001–8,000	2,101–2,400	17
8,001–9,000	2,401–2,700	18
9,001–10,000	2,701–3,000	19

BLACKBERRY-INFUSED VINEGAR

This recipe should work well with similar wild berries such as mulberries, raspberries, boysenberries, dewberries, currants, and so on. It's pretty much identical to the Blueberry-Mugwort-Infused Vinegar process aside from the fact that we boil the berries with the vinegar instead of crushing them, but you can use the blueberry method if desired.

Ingredients for a 1-quart jar (1 L)

2 cups (12 ounces, or 340 g) blackberries

Optional flavorings: I've made this flavored vinegar using all kinds of wild savory herbs, such as California sagebrush, yarrow, and mugwort (usually 2 to 3 leaves). A small, cracked pinyon pine branch (3 to 4 inches, or 7.5 to 10 cm) placed in the cold vinegar imbued a wonderful savory accent. Commercial savory herbs could include basil, fennel, or dill.

2 cups (480 ml) red or white wine vinegar (apple cider vinegar works great, too)

Procedure

Rinse the blackberries briefly under cold running water, making sure to remove any rotten berries. Place the berries and flavorings of your choice into a nonreactive pot (stainless steel or enamel coated), then add the vinegar. Bring the contents to boil, then reduce the heat and simmer for around 3 to 4 minutes. You can simmer for a shorter time when using tender berries such as raspberries.

Transfer the contents into a quart (1 L) jar. Cap tightly and place in a cool, dark place for 2 to 3 weeks. I like to shake the jar once a week.

Strain and transfer the vinegar into clean bottles or a pint (480 ml) jar. Seal tightly and store in the refrigerator or a cool, dark place (below 65°F/18°C). Shelf life for optimum flavors is around 6 months, or up to a year in perfect storage conditions.

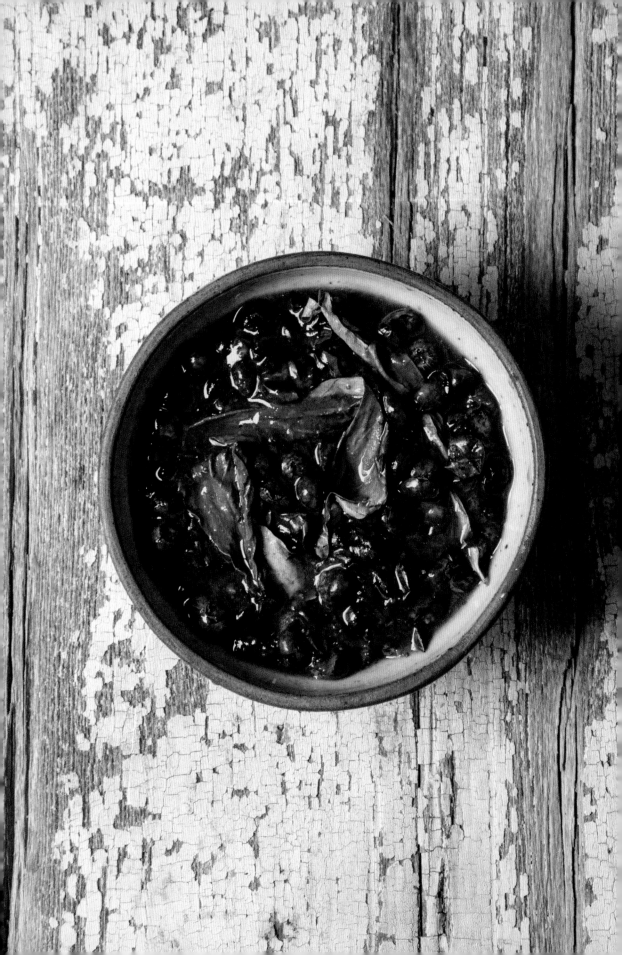

BLUEBERRY-MUGWORT-INFUSED VINEGAR

There are several methods for making vinegars flavored with berries. They are similar and somewhat interchangeable. To infuse with unusual wild berries, take a look at the various recipes in this chapter and choose one that seems appropriate based on the berry types. For example, wild currants would work well in Blackcurrant-Infused Vinegar. Where I lived in Southern California, I made some coffeeberry vinegar using the recipe for blueberry-mugwort vinegar, as the texture of the berries is somewhat similar.

My favorite homemade or wildcrafted vinegars to use for this recipe are Prickly Pear Lazy Wine Vinegar or Elderberry Wine Vinegar. Some store-bought blueberries can be quite tasteless—it's hard to beat the flavors of wild blueberries picked at their prime.

Ingredients for a 1-quart jar (1 L)

2 cups (12 ounces, or 340 g) fresh or frozen blueberries

Optional flavorings: 2 to 3 dried mugwort leaves or a couple of dried yarrow flower heads (or leaves) or your own wildcrafted herbs

2 cups (480 ml) red or white wine vinegar

2 to 3 tablespoons (30–45 ml) maple syrup (or honey or sugar)

Procedure

Rinse the blueberries briefly under cold running water, making sure to remove any rotten berries. In a nonreactive container, crush the blueberries using a fork, spoon, or potato masher. You can also use your (clean) hands if you want—blueberries don't tint your skin very much. It should take a minute or so. You're not trying to make a puree; you simply want to break the berries so the flavors can imbue the vinegar. Transfer the crushed berries to a quart (1 L) jar and add the flavoring leaves (mugwort, yarrow, or wildcrafted herbs).

Heat the vinegar and maple syrup to just below boiling, then pour the mixture into the jar. Cap tightly and place in a cool, dark place for 2 to 3 weeks. I like to shake the jar once a week.

Strain and transfer the vinegar into clean bottles or a pint (480 ml) jar. Seal tightly and store in the refrigerator or another cool, dark place (below 65°F/18°C). Shelf life for optimum flavors is around 6 months and up to a year in perfect storage conditions.

ELDERBERRY-INFUSED VINEGAR

This could be my favorite vinegar. I've made a lot of Elderberry Wine Vinegar, and while it's quite good, the flavors of infused, dehydrated berries are hard to beat. You can use a good homemade or commercial vinegar to make this, but . . . come on! You can't beat elderberries infused in elderberry wine!

The method is similar to that of Blackberry-Infused Vinegar. Elderberries should be cooked prior to consumption, so we'll boil and simmer them a bit.

Ingredients for a 1-pint jar (480 ml)

¼ cup (1 ounce, or 28 g) dried elderberries
2 cups (480 ml) red wine vinegar
   or Elderberry Wine Vinegar, divided

Procedure

Place the dried berries in a nonreactive pot and add 1 cup (240 ml) of the vinegar. Bring the contents to boil for 3 minutes, then reduce the heat, add the rest of the vinegar, and simmer for another 3 minutes.

Transfer the contents into a pint (480 ml) jar. Cap tightly and place in a cool, dark place for 2 to 3 weeks. I like to shake the jar once a week.

Strain and transfer the vinegar into clean bottles or a fresh pint (480 ml) jar. Seal tightly and store in the refrigerator or a cool, dark place (below 65°F/18°C). Shelf life for optimum flavors is around 6 months, or up to a year in perfect storage conditions.

BLACKCURRANT-INFUSED VINEGAR

This vinegar is fantastic with store-bought blackcurrants (*Ribes nigrum*), which are also called cassis. Sadly, the currants I collect locally, golden currants (*R. aureum*), don't have the same intense flavor.

This recipe works better with less sugar than usual. Some traditional recipes for blackcurrant vinegar will ask for much more sugar—up to 3 times the amount listed here—and 1 stick of cinnamon as flavoring. The resulting sweet fruit vinegar is used in sauces, salad dressings, and desserts, or diluted to make a refreshing drink.

Ingredients for a 1-quart jar (1 L)

17 ounces (482 g) blackcurrants

2 cups (480 ml) red wine vinegar

¼ cup (60 ml) maple syrup or 5 ounces (140 g) granulated sugar

Procedure

Rinse the blackcurrant berries briefly under cold running water, making sure to remove any rotten berries. In a nonreactive container, crush the berries using a fork, spoon, or potato masher. It should take a minute or so. You're not trying to make a puree; you simply want to break the berries so the flavors can imbue the vinegar. Transfer the crushed berries into a quart (1 L) jar.

Heat the vinegar and maple syrup to just below boiling, then pour it inside the jar. Cap tightly and place in a cool, dark place for 2 to 3 weeks. I like to shake the jar once a week.

Strain and transfer the vinegar into clean bottles or a pint (480 ml) jar. Seal tightly and store in the refrigerator or a cool, dark place (below 65°F/18°C). Shelf life for optimum flavors is around 6 months.

RAW INFUSION OF BERRIES
IN UNPASTEURIZED VINEGAR

Some people (like me) want to keep the probiotics and fresh taste of raw ingredients, but most of the recipes for flavoring vinegars with berries ask for heating the vinegar, which kills the yeast and other bacteria (including *Acetobacter*) present on the berries. Heating also alters the flavors.

Based on what I've read, the recommendation to heat seems to come from the possibility of wild yeast fermentation occurring. This doesn't make a lot of sense to me, as eventually the fermentation would become vinegar anyway. Without heating, there is also the possibility that unwanted bacteria could spoil the vinegar or create mold. A buildup of bacteria is not an issue, as the pH of vinegar is too low (meaning it's acidic). Berries are usually quite acidic, too, so the whole infusion is safe for consumption.

You can find recipes online for making raw infused vinegars, and I've followed a lot of them with great success. I can understand that, from a commercial perspective, pasteurizing the vinegar is a necessity because you don't know if the vinegar will be properly stored and for how long. But if you make vinegar for personal consumption, you can take care of your raw infusion and store it properly.

My only advice is to toss the contents if you see any mold or signs of spoilage (bad smell, slime, and so on). It's also important to shake the contents at least once a day for the first week. This will distribute the acidity and inhibit the possibility of mold growing on the surface.

Ingredients for a 1-pint jar (480 ml)

6 ounces (170 g) organic blackberries, blueberries, or the like

Optional flavorings: basil, wild tarragon, mugwort, and so forth

3 tablespoons (45 ml) maple syrup

1½ cups (360 ml) unpasteurized red wine vinegar

Procedure

Inspect the berries for freshness and quality, tossing any with mold. Remove the stems, then place the berries in a colander and wash in cold water. Clean any herbs you want to use as additional flavoring and bruise them a bit, which will help extract the flavors.

Transfer the berries to a bowl and crush them into a rough pulp with a fork or your (clean) hands. You can also use a blender. Transfer the contents into a clean or pasteurized pint jar. Add the maple syrup and pour the vinegar over the berries.

Cap tightly and place in a cool, dark place for around 2 weeks. I like to shake the jar once a week.

Strain the vinegar into a new jar and store in the fridge. For optimum flavors and food safety, I don't age raw infused vinegars for more than a couple of months.

ROOTS VINEGAR: AMERICAN LICORICE

This basic recipe should work with other savory roots, such as sarsaparilla or sassafras, although you may need to adjust the quantity. In this recipe I use dehydrated licorice roots, but I don't see why you couldn't use fresh roots. The roots are heated with the vinegar to facilitate flavor extraction.

Ingredients for a 1-pint jar (480 ml)

0.7 ounces (20 g) dehydrated American licorice (*Glycyrrhiza lepidota*) root

1¾ cups (420 ml) apple cider vinegar

4 teaspoons (20 ml) maple syrup, sugar, or honey

Procedure

Clean the licorice roots thoroughly to remove any remaining dirt and cut them into small pieces of around 1 inch (2.5 cm) in length.

Heat the vinegar with the roots and maple syrup to just below boiling, then simmer for 3 to 4 minutes. Pour the mixture into a pint jar. Cap tightly and place in a cool, dark place for 3 to 4 weeks. I like to shake the jar once a week.

Taste the vinegar. If you're not satisfied with the flavors, you can age the vinegar and roots for another 3 weeks before straining. If you are satisfied, strain and transfer into clean bottles or a pint jar. Seal tightly and store in the refrigerator or a cool, dark place (below 65°F/18°C). Shelf life for optimum flavors is around 6 months, or up to a year in perfect storage conditions.

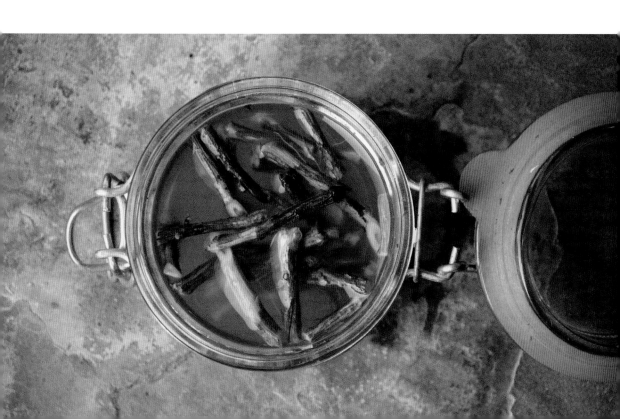

Herb and Stem Vinegars

You'll find tons of recipes for herbal vinegars online and in books, but when it comes to wild herbs, you'll probably need to experiment quite a bit. Where I lived in Southern California, some of the local savory and aromatic wild herbs were so strong that making these types of vinegars was truly an exercise in moderation.

So don't get discouraged if your first attempts using local wild ingredients do not turn out very well. I learned a lot from my mistakes. With experience you can truly make some incredible gourmet vinegars.

You can start by experimenting with commercial herbs. The most common ones used to infuse vinegars are dill, basil, rosemary, tarragon, fennel, thyme, lemongrass, parsley, bay leaves, lemon zest, garlic, lavender, chives, and mustard seeds.

Some of the local wild aromatic plants I've used to infuse vinegars include California sagebrush, mugwort, wild tarragon, yarrow, California bay, sweet white clover, black mustard seeds, pine and fir needles, oak bark, mesquite, juniper berries, various sages, wild fennel, water mint, wild rose hips, manzanita berries, elderflowers, pineapple weed (*Matricaria discoidea*), and more.

Aside from herbs, I also like to infuse with aromatic stems. When I dehydrate my herbs for various purposes, I usually keep the stems. The stems can be used to flavor soups, make sodas, infuse flavors into ferments, and more. You can even make interesting blends by using the stems from various plants.

Although you will find variations in traditional infused-vinegar recipes, the basic guidelines from various government agencies on ratios of ingredients to 2 cups (480 ml) vinegar are as follows:

> 3 to 4 sprigs
> or
> ½ cup (25 g) bruised fresh herbs
> or
> 1 to 3 tablespoons (9–18 g) dried herbs

While this is a good starting point, the reality is sometimes quite different. For example, 1 tablespoon (9 g) of dried California sagebrush in 2 cups (480 ml) of vinegar will result in a disgustingly bitter and unusable vinegar. One small, fresh sprig is more than enough. Sagebrush is usually used in tiny amounts in combination with other herbs or spices.

You can blend ingredients, too. For example, here are the ingredients for a recipe from the Colorado State University Extension:

Herbal Vinegar

4 cups red wine vinegar
8 sprigs fresh parsley
2 teaspoons thyme leaves
1 teaspoon rosemary leaves
1 teaspoon sage leaves*

It's also very common to pair herbs with spices. Good pairings, for example, are tarragon with garlic, or dill with dried red peppers. One of my favorites is vinegar infused with wild tarragon and black mustard seeds. You can also season the infused vinegar with sugar or salt.

Distilled white vinegar is often used for infusing herbs and stems, as it is quite neutral in flavor, but I prefer to use apple cider vinegar or my own homemade vinegars. It is recommended to use vinegar with a minimum of 5 percent acidity.

Of course, the ability to make your own vinegar will open a new universe of flavors. A big part of the fun is the creative pairing of vinegar and the ingredients used to flavor the vinegar. My homemade perry (fermented pears) vinegar infused with white fir needles is truly a divine pairing.

Methods of Infusion

For herbs and stems, I decide which infusion method (hot or cold) to use strictly based on flavors. You will have more success extracting flavor from some herbs—such as thyme and mugwort—using the Hot Method Procedure; while other herbs—such as pineapple weed, basil, and mint—will fare much better with the Cold Method Procedure that follows. I don't use the Hot Method Procedure for pine, fir, spruce needles, or juniper berries, as doing so alters the flavors too much.

HOT METHOD PROCEDURE

Pour the amount of vinegar you want to use into a nonreactive pot, and start by heating it to just below boiling.

While the vinegar is heating, clean and lightly bruise the herbs you want to use. This will help release their essence. You can do this using your fingers or by placing the herbs on a clean cutting board and pressing them with the

---

* D. Grubb, E. Shackleton, and M. Bunning, "Making Flavored Vinegar—9.340," Colorado State University Extension, January 2021, https://extension.colostate .edu/topic-areas/nutrition-food-safety-health/flavored-vinegars-and-oils-9-340/.

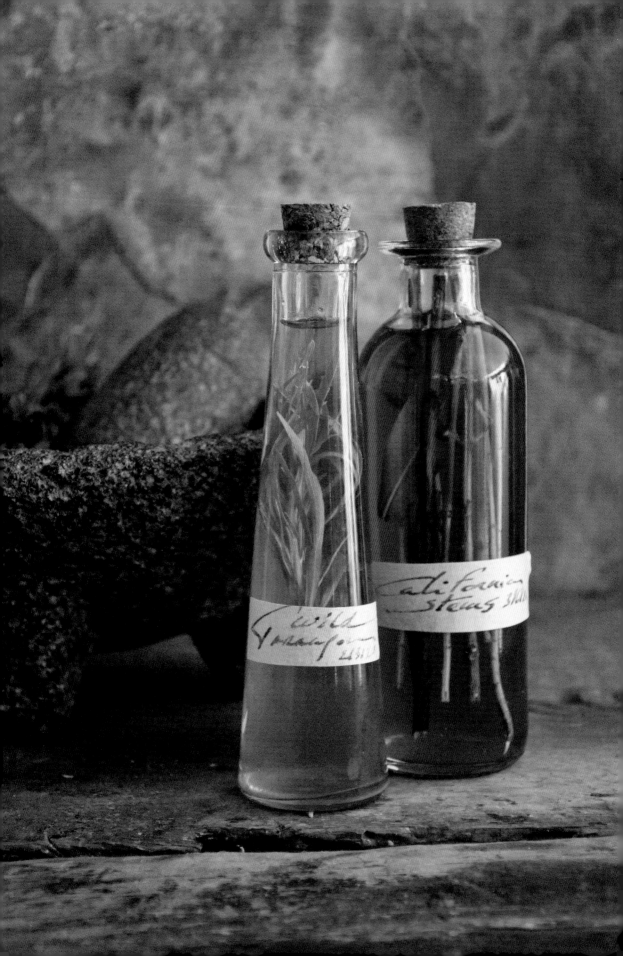

back of a spoon. You can also use a mortar and pestle, but remember that the idea is to bruise slightly.

Place the herbs and any additional spices in a glass jar or similar container, then pour the heated vinegar over the ingredients. Leave ¼ inch (0.6 cm) headspace and seal tightly.

Store in a cool, dark place for around 10 days, then taste. If you like the flavors, strain and bottle the vinegar. Otherwise, you can age it longer, usually up to 3 to 4 weeks. If you think the flavors are too strong, you can dilute the infused vinegar by adding more heated vinegar.

Once bottled, cap tightly and store in the refrigerator or a cool, dark place (below 65°F/18°C). Shelf life for optimum flavors is around 6 months, or up to a year in perfect storage conditions.

COLD METHOD PROCEDURE

Clean and lightly bruise the herbs you want to use as with hot method then place them in a glass jar or bottle. For pine or fir needles, you will need to cut the needle tips to facilitate flavor extraction. Coarsely chopping will also work for herbs such as mint or basil.

Cover the ingredients with room-temperature vinegar. Leave ¼ inch (0.6 cm) headspace and seal tightly.

Store in a cool, dark place for around 10 days, then taste. If you like the flavor, strain and bottle the vinegar. Otherwise, you can age it longer, usually up to 3 to 4 weeks. If you think the flavors are too strong, you can dilute the infused vinegar by adding more room-temperature vinegar. Based on personal experience, pine and fir needles benefit from a much longer infusing period—weeks or sometimes months.

Once bottled, cap tightly and store in the refrigerator or a cool, dark place (below 65°F/18°C). Shelf life for optimum flavors is around 6 months, or up to a year in perfect storage conditions.

Vinegars infused with wild tarragon and local aromatic stems.

ELDERFLOWER-INFUSED VINEGAR

So delicious and yet so easy to make. Each year I make a batch of this vinegar with elderflowers from local Mexican elder (*Sambucus mexicana*), which I think are a bit milder than black elder (*S. nigra*) with their own flavor accents. This is a classic recipe in Europe and particularly England.

When foraging elderflowers, you want them full of pollen. The newly opened flowers are best. Collect them in the morning on a sunny day and place them into a paper bag.

It's common to have a lot of tiny flies present on the flowers. My method of getting rid of them is to place the flowers in a bowl outside for an hour or so. Most of the little critters will vacate. Another technique is to gently shake the flowers. Don't run the flowers under water, as you'll wash off the pollen and much of the flavors.

Ingredients for a 1-pint jar (480 ml)

Around 10 elderflower heads from Mexican elder, or 4 to 5 elderflower heads from black elder

2 to 3 tablespoons (30 to 45 ml) maple syrup (optional at this stage—you can season the vinegar later, too)

1¾ cups (420 ml) apple cider vinegar (raw or pasteurized), see Note

Note: You can also use white wine, rice, or champagne vinegar for this recipe.

Procedure

Use the flowers as soon as possible after harvesting. To remove them from the stalk and small stems, rub gently with your thumb and forefinger in a downward motion over a bowl. They should drop without much effort. It's harder to do if you wait too long and the flower heads are slightly wilted.

The size of the flowers will vary based on the type of elder tree, but the idea is to pack them very loosely into the pint jar.

Add the maple syrup and vinegar, then close the lid. Shake the jar gently so the syrup and vinegar mix well. You want the jar to be quite full—you can add more vinegar if necessary.

Let stand for 2 to 3 weeks in a cool, dark place. Strain the vinegar and discard the flowers. Transfer the vinegar into a clean bottle or glass container. Cap tightly and store in the refrigerator or a cool, dark place (below 65°F/18°C). Shelf life for optimum flavors is around 6 months, or up to a year in perfect storage conditions.

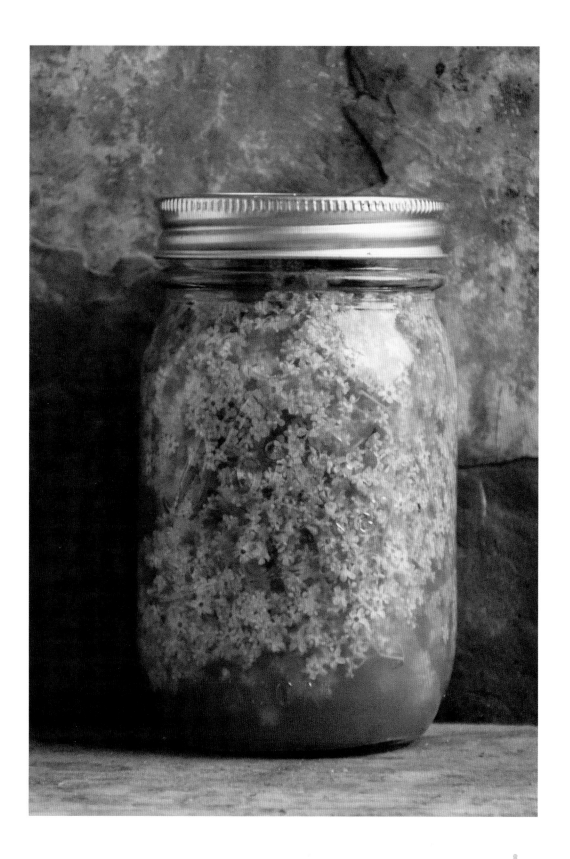

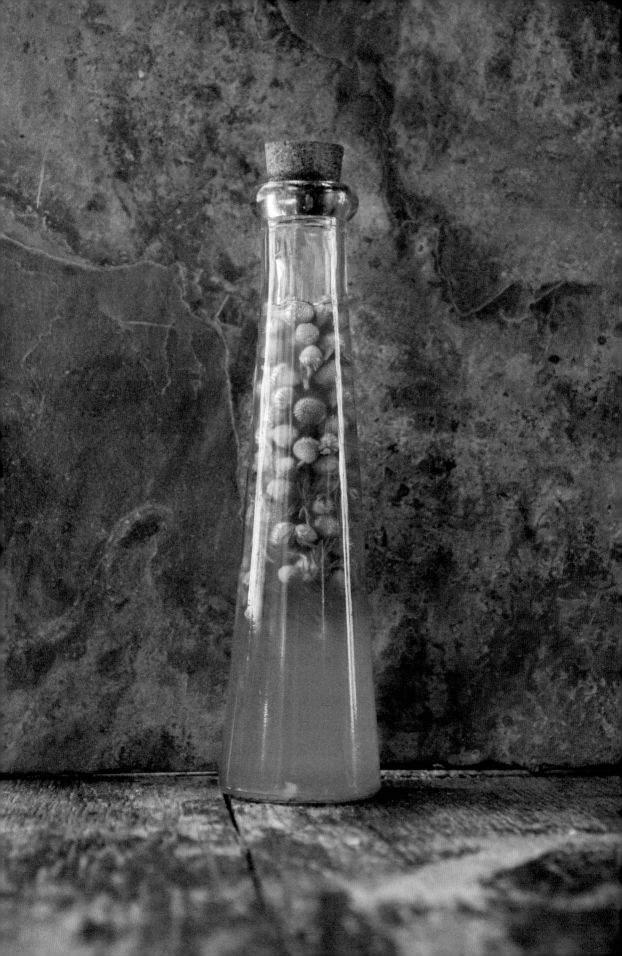

PINEAPPLE WEED–INFUSED VINEGAR

Pineapple weed is perhaps better known as chamomile. You can make this recipe with wild or regular varieties of this plant. Although the flavors won't be the same, both will result in a delicious vinegar. The plant I forage locally is called pineapple weed for good reason: The flowers taste very much like pineapple. It does not have the white petals often associated with chamomile flowers, however.

Pineapple weed is an annual plant native to northeast Asia, but you'll find it all over North America, Canada, and England. I find it on hiking trails, along roadsides, and in city parks and construction areas. The plant loves disturbed soil.

When you forage it, make sure you're not in an area where herbicides are sprayed. As its name indicates, it's considered a weed. I've always been able to find pristine locations to forage it. In Los Angeles, I used to find it on the hiking trails in the Angeles National Forest. I'm currently in Colorado and visited a friend who is an organic farmer. The plant was quite abundant on his property.

I only use the flowers, which are easy to remove. I don't bother collecting the leaves, as they don't have much flavor. For making the infused vinegar, its best to use the flowers fresh for optimal flavor.

I've never bothered weighing the flowers for a recipe. I've always used the ratio of 1 part flower heads to 2 parts vinegar.

Ingredients for a 1-cup jar (240 ml)

⅓ cup (17 g) pineapple weed flowers

⅔ cup (160 ml) apple cider vinegar (raw or pasteurized), see Note

2½ tablespoons (37 ml) maple syrup

1½ teaspoons (7.5 g) salt

Note: *A good quality organic and unpasteurized vinegar will work nicely. I usually use my own homemade Apple Scraps Vinegar or Mugwort Beer Vinegar. Based on the recipe, this is more like a seasoned vinegar— you can skip the maple syrup and salt if you want.*

Procedure

Rinse the flowers briefly under cold running water, then place them in a jar, bottle, or similar glass container. Mix the vinegar, maple syrup, and salt together. Pour the seasoned vinegar over the flowers. Fill the container as much as possible, minimizing the amount of oxygen.

Cap tightly and allow to stand 2 to 3 weeks in a cool, dark place. Strain the vinegar and discard the flowers. Transfer the vinegar into a clean bottle or glass container. Seal tightly and store in the refrigerator or a cool, dark place (below 65°F/18°C). Shelf life for optimum flavors is around 6 months, or up to a year in perfect storage conditions.

FRESH HERBAL-INFUSED VINEGARS

Making a fresh herbal vinegar is something I often did right after a plant identification walk with my students. I would simply collect herbs along with other savory ingredients during the walk, then place them in a pint jar with 1 cup (240 ml) of homemade vinegar. Next, using a handheld blender, I would create a beautiful and tasty vinegar on location. These vinegars were then used as a base to make wild food salad dressings.

Typical wildcrafted herbs would include chickweed, sweet cicely (*Myrrhis odorata*) roots, wild chervil, miner's lettuce (*Claytonia perfoliata*), grass, wild carrots (*Daucus carota*), oxalis, pineapple weed, and so on. Of course, you can do something similar with store-bought ingredients such as parsley, cilantro, basil, and other herbs.

Ingredients for a 1-pint jar (480 ml)

Around 1 ounce (28 g) freshly foraged (or commercial) herbs
1 cup (240 ml) unpasteurized Apple Scraps Vinegar

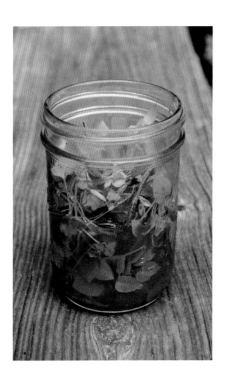

Procedure

Place your herbs and any other collected ingredients you want to use in a large-mouth jar, then add the vinegar. Your other option is to place everything into a regular blender (instead of using a handheld blender in the jar).

Blend the ingredients and strain the herbal vinegar into a bottle. You're done!

This is something you need to use right away if you want to keep the beautiful green color. It usually turns tan or brownish within 30 minutes, which I personally don't mind.

When you find the right combination of herbs, this type of vinegar is really packed with flavors.

Salad Dressing

Feel free to get creative with this base recipe and make a good salad dressing on the spot. For example, before blending, try adding the following ingredients:

2 tablespoons (30 ml) maple syrup
1½ teaspoons (7.5 g) salt
1 ounce (28 g) minced jalapeños (optional)
1 minced garlic clove
0.5 ounce (14 g) chopped red onions
0.5 ounce (14 g) fresh ginger

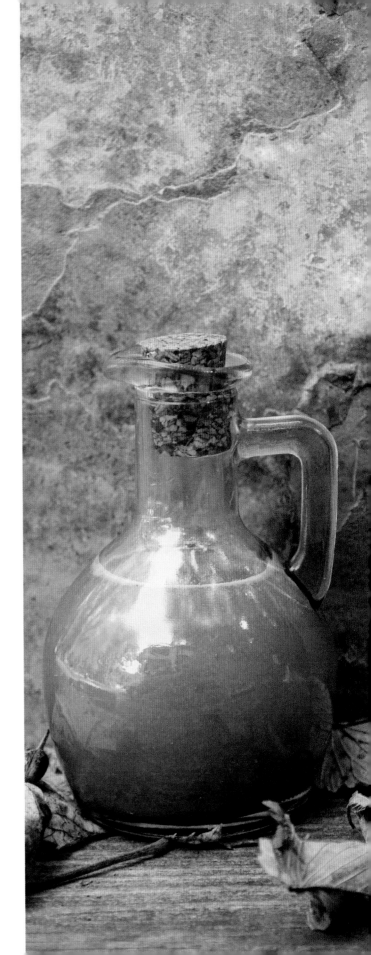

PINE-, FIR-, AND SPRUCE-INFUSED VINEGARS

You can make truly delicious vinegars by infusing pine, fir, or spruce needles. All species in the *Pinus* genus are "edible," but don't get all excited yet. Not all *Pinus* needles will taste great. Some are bitter or tasteless, while others are extremely flavorful. Most people think that pine needles taste like "pine," but they're usually quite lemony and can have tangerine-like flavors.

The best way to test is to grab a couple of needles and chew—if they taste great, you're good to go! Common pines I've used so far include white pine (*Pinus strobus*), ponderosa pine, and pinyon pine.

Other trees that I've used for this recipe are Douglas fir (*Pseudotsuga menziesii*), spruce tips from Engelmann spruce (*Picea engelmannii*), Colorado blue spruce (*Picea pungens*), and white fir.

Be aware that some trees look like pines but are not from the *Pinus* genus. They can be quite toxic. Examples include the Norfolk Island pine and yew. As any wildcrafter knows, you need to properly ID and research any plant you use.

Ingredients for a 1-pint jar (480 ml)

Enough pine needles, spruce tips, or small white fir branches to (very) loosely fill three-quarters of the jar (see Note)

1½ cups (360 ml) apple cider vinegar or other vinegar

3 tablespoons (45 ml) maple syrup, honey, or sugar (optional)

1½ teaspoons (7.5 g) salt (optional)

Procedure

Chop the needles or cut their tips (spruce or fir) to help extract the flavors. Loosely pack a clean pint (480 ml) jar with the needles you want to use—three-quarters full is perfect.

Mix the vinegar, maple syrup, and salt together. (You can skip the sugar and salt, but I think this vinegar is much better when seasoned.) Pour the seasoned vinegar into the jar containing the pine needles, spruce tips, or fir. Close the jar and store for at least 6 weeks in a cool, dark place.

Taste. If it's too strong you can add more vinegar. Strain and transfer the vinegar into a clean bottle or glass container. Seal tightly and store in the refrigerator or a cool, dark place (below 65°F/18°C). Shelf life for optimum flavors is up to a couple of years in perfect storage conditions.

*Note: It is not advised to consume pine, fir, or spruce if you are pregnant. I know we're using small quantities, but some pines, such as ponderosa pine, may have some abortive qualities. **Do not** make vinegar with any purchased Christmas tree. They are often sprayed with chemicals to keep longer.*

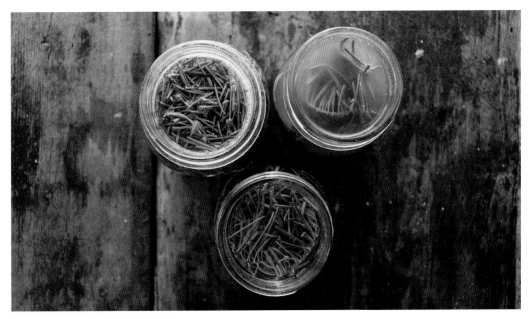

Clockwise, starting from the bottom: Pinyon pine–, ponderosa pine–, and white fir–infused vinegars.

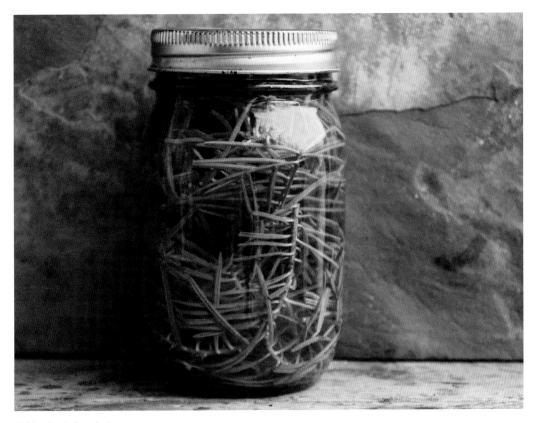

White fir–infused vinegar.

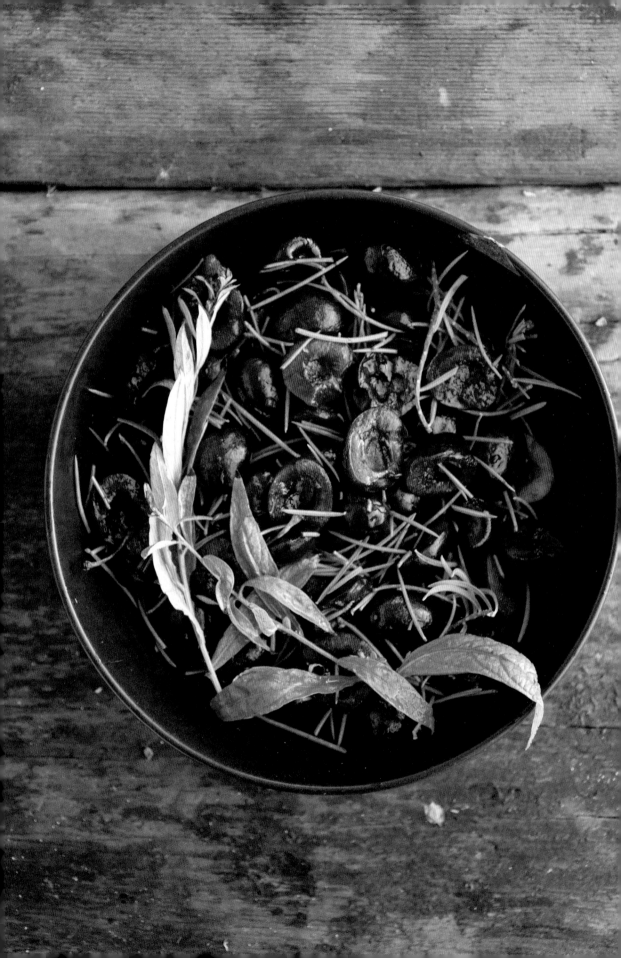

CHERRY, MUGWORT, WHITE FIR, AND PINYON PINE–INFUSED VINEGAR

Not everything in your vinegar has to be wild. I often use commercial fruits and berries but add savory wild plants to bring the flavors to a new level. Mugwort is one of my favorite plants to use to bring a sort of umami flavor to sweet concoctions. In this case, the bitterness of the mugwort is balanced by the sweetness of the fully ripe cherries, and you get the benefit of the wonderful aromatics that mugwort can offer. Pinyon pine and white fir needles add tangerine, lemony, and pine accents.

For most of my berry-infused vinegars, I use a ratio of around 40 percent berries to 60 percent vinegar (at 5 percent acidity).

The recipe is straightforward—note that for cherries I remove the pits, which contains some cyanide. Honestly, I have no idea if that could leach into the vinegar. Better safe than sorry. I use the "Cold Method Procedure" (page 93). You could heat the vinegar, but too much heat will alter the pine/fir flavors.

Ingredients for a 1-quart jar (1 L)

2 cups (380 g) cherries
1 teaspoon (2 g) white fir needles
1 tablespoon (5 g) pinyon pine needles
2⅓ cups (560 ml) raw apple cider
    or red wine vinegar (see Note)
2 tablespoons (30 ml) maple syrup
1 teaspoon (5 g) sea salt
2 mugwort sprigs

Note: *Instead of apple cider or red wine vinegar, I often use my Elderberry Wine Vinegar.*

Procedure

Rinse the cherries briefly under cold running water, making sure to remove any rotten ones. Cut each cherry in two and remove the pit. Transfer the cherries to a quart jar.

Chop or cut the white fir and pine needles and add them to the jar.

Add the remaining ingredients to the jar, leaving around ¾ inch (2 cm) headspace.

Due to the sugar and wild yeast present on the ingredients, expect some active fermentation during the first week or two. My method is to open the jar briefly a couple of times daily and stir the contents. If you still notice excessive pressure, burp the jar (unscrew the top to reduce pressure).

When the fermentation is complete (no more fermentation gases), you can close the jar, then store it for at least another 4 weeks in a cool, dark place.

Strain and transfer the infused vinegar into a clean bottle or glass container. Seal tightly and store in the refrigerator or a cool, dark place (below 65°F/18°C). Shelf life for optimum flavors is around 6 months, or up to a year in perfect storage conditions.

PRICKLY PEAR–INFUSED VINEGAR WITH MUGWORT, WHITE FIR, AND PINYON PINE NEEDLES

This recipe is nearly identical to the Cherry, Mugwort, White Fir, and Pinyon Pine–Infused Vinegar recipe, but in this case, everything can be foraged. You can purchase prickly pears at Hispanic supermarkets, but I find that the ones I collect in nature are much tastier if picked at their prime. The flavor reminds me of a super sweet watermelon.

My wild prickly pears are one-third the size of the commercial ones and contain many more seeds. Instead of cutting them, I use a knife and stab them around 6 to 8 times so the flavors can be extracted. I also find that this technique makes my vinegar less mucilaginous, or sticky, than if I cut them.

Ingredients for a 1-quart jar (1 L)

Enough prickly pears to fill three-quarters of a quart (1 L) jar (see Note)

2 cups (480 ml) raw apple cider vinegar (if you need a bit more to fill the jar, go ahead)

1 teaspoon (2 g) white fir needles

1 tablespoon (5 g) pinyon pine needles

2 tablespoons (30 ml) maple syrup

1 teaspoon (5 g) sea salt

1 mugwort sprig

Procedure

Rinse the prickly pears briefly under cold running water, making sure to remove any rotten ones. Stab each pear 6 to 8 times with a knife, then transfer the pears to a quart (1 L) jar. Although the jar will be filled with pears, you'll notice lots of space between them, which will be filled by the vinegar.

Chop or cut the fir and pine needles in two.

Place all the ingredients in the jar, leaving around ¾ inch (2 cm) headspace. For the first 2 weeks, I don't close the jar but secure a paper towel on top and stir the contents once a day. You can also close the jar, shake the contents, and burp it if any fermentation is occurring.

After 2 weeks, remove the paper towel and close the jar, then store it for at least another 4 weeks in a cool, dark place. Strain and transfer the infused vinegar into a clean bottle or glass container. Seal tightly and store in the refrigerator or a cool, dark place (below 65°F/18°C). Shelf life for optimum flavors is around 6 months, or up to a year with good storage.

> **Note:** If I use commercial prickly pears for this recipe, which are much bigger, I use a 1-gallon jar and adapt the recipe accordingly (four times larger). You could also slice the commercial prickly pears instead of stabbing them so they will fit in the smaller jar.

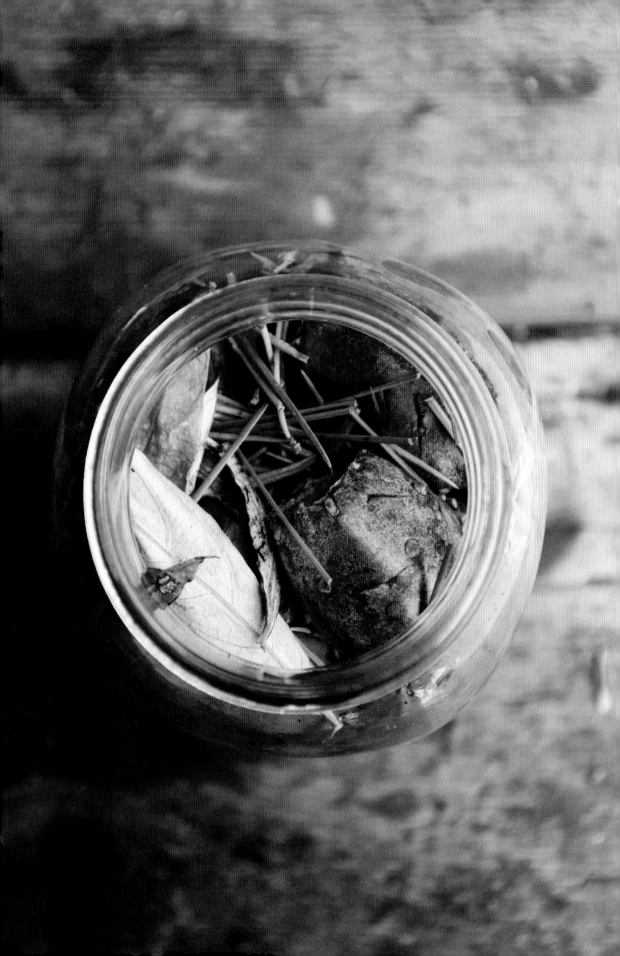

PINYON PINE–INFUSED VINEGAR

You don't need many ingredients to make this infused vinegar, and it's absolutely awesome. When I was living in Southern California, I would often visit my friend Gloria who has a goat farm in the local mountains. Her beautiful property is mostly composed of pinyon pines and California junipers.

My main forages at her property were pinyon pine nuts, California juniper berries, and unripe pinyon pine cones, which I would use for pine cone syrup or as a source of wild yeast. While foraging the pine cones, I would always end up with some pine sap on my hands. I could not get enough of the perfume emanating from the sap. It had the sweetness of candy and hints of tangerine and pine.

Of course, I had to try it, but chewing the sap was a less delightful experience. It was slightly bitter and would stick to my teeth. But I never gave up, and my eureka moment occurred while I was picking up an unripe pinyon pine cone and broke a branch while doing it. The smell inside the pinyon branch was even better than the sap, which gave me an idea. . . . What if I infused some small, broken pinyon branches into vinegar?

As soon as I arrived home, I cracked some branches in two and placed them in vinegar for around 3 weeks. I totally fell in love with the result. It didn't have the bitterness you find in the sap. To this day, it's one of the best vinegars I've made. Here is the basic recipe I use; you can skip the sugar if desired, as the vinegar will have some sweetness from the pine. You can also add the sugar later on in the process if you decide you want it.

Ingredients for a 1-quart jar (1 L)

Enough cracked pinyon pine branches to loosely fill around one-half of a quart (1 L) jar (see Note)

3¼ cups (780 ml) pasteurized apple cider vinegar

5 tablespoons (75 ml) maple syrup, honey, or sugar (2.2 ounces, or 62 g)

Note: Based on experience, for optimum flavors you want to forage the branches in late spring and early summer.

Procedure

Use a good pruning shear or small handsaw for this recipe. We're just making a quart jar, so you don't need much. You're looking for small pinyon pine branches that are around 4 inches (10 cm) in length and ½ inch (1.3 cm) in diameter. Cut a branch, remove the small branches and needles connected to it, and place the small branches in a bag. Keep going until you have enough to fill half of the jar you plan to use.

Use the branches as soon as possible, preferably within 24 to 48 hours. Thoroughly clean your branches in cold water. I use a scrub brush. To release the flavors, split the branches in two, lengthwise. You can make an incision at one end with a pruning shear and open it with your fingers.

Place the split branches into the jar and add the vinegar and maple syrup. Don't heat the vinegar, as it will alter the flavors. Cap tightly and place in cool, dark place. Shake the contents at least once a day for the first 10 days. Age for around 2 months.

Strain and transfer the vinegar into clean bottles or similar glass containers. Seal tightly and store in the refrigerator or a cool, dark place. This will taste awesome for years.

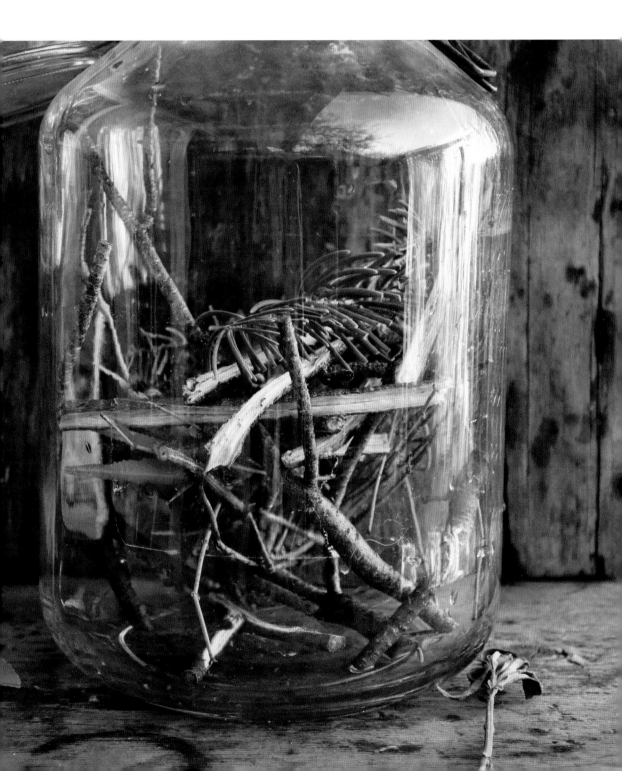

SEAWEED-INFUSED VINEGAR

This is truly one of my favorite vinegars. You immediately think of the sea when you taste it, and it's so easy to make. This recipe uses wakame and kombu, which can be wildcrafted from the coastlines of California or purchased at Asian food stores. If you're a seaweed forager, feel free to experiment with your local seaweed.

Ingredients for a 1-quart jar (1 L)

4 to 5 tablespoons (60 to 75 ml) maple syrup
0.7 ounces (20 g) dried kelp (kombu)
0.7 ounces (20 g) wakame
2 chili pods (mild or spicy)
1½ to 2 tablespoons (22.5 to 30 g) sea salt
1 teaspoon (3 g) whole peppercorns
3½ cups (840 ml) apple cider vinegar or rice vinegar (see Note)

Procedure

Combine all the ingredients except the vinegar in a quart (1 L) jar. Heat the vinegar to just below the boiling point, then pour into the jar. Cap tightly and place in a cool, dark place for 2 to 3 weeks. I shake the jar a couple of times each week.

Strain and transfer the vinegar into clean bottles or similar glass containers. Seal tightly and store in the refrigerator or a cool, dark place (below 65°F/18°C). Shelf life for optimum flavors is around 6 months, or up to a year in perfect storage conditions.

> **Note:** I've also made this recipe with raw vinegar, and it worked fine. The flavors were stronger with the heated vinegar. If you have a kitchen smoker, try this recipe with smoked seaweed. It's delicious (see also Smoked Mushrooms and Seaweed–Infused Vinegar).

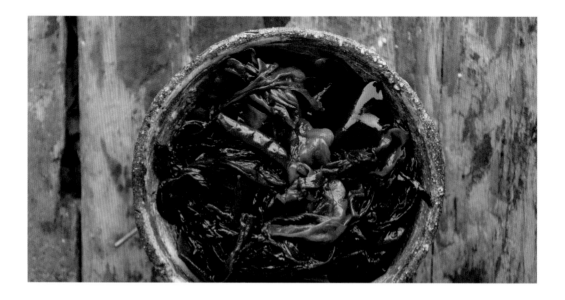

SMOKED MUSHROOM-INFUSED VINEGAR

During a good year, I often have a surplus of mushrooms. Last year this was the case with oyster mushrooms. In order not to waste this precious resource, I use many methods of food preservation—dehydration, freezing, fermenting, and so on.

But sometimes it's not just about eating mushrooms—you can also think of them as a potential flavor additive. This is exactly what we're doing by creating a delicious infused vinegar. Of course, to make such vinegar, the choice of mushrooms is key. In this case I used commercial shiitake and some of my very fragrant wild oyster mushrooms. I would have added a couple of candy caps, but I had used them all already.

I always use dehydrated mushrooms for making this infusion; I think they are more pungent. Aside from mushrooms, the next savory layer comes from smoking the mushrooms before infusing. You can go hyperlocal in your choice of flavorful woods and plants. For this recipe I use a blend of oak bark, mesquite wood, and rabbit tobacco (*Pseudognaphalium canescens*), which has a curry flavor. The bark and wood were collected from fallen trees.

This procedure is very similar to the Smoked Mushrooms and Seaweed–Infused Vinegar.

Ingredients for a 1-quart jar (1 L)

1.7 ounces (45 g) dried savory mushrooms
   (commercial shiitake, wild oyster, or others)
Commercial or foraged wood chips, barks,
   or herbs (for smoking), see Note
2½ cups (600 ml) raw apple cider vinegar
5 tablespoons (75 ml) maple syrup or honey
2½ teaspoon (12.5 g) salt

Note: Wood chips for smoking, such as mesquite, apple, hickory, can be found in large supermarkets or purchased online. You can purchase handheld kitchen smokers online. Search for "smoke infusers," "handheld smoker," or "smoking gun." The brand name of the one I use is HANDi SMoK.

Procedure

Place the mushrooms in a quart (1 L) jar, close the smoker lid on it, and attach the handheld smoker. Insert your wood and herbs in the smoker and smoke the contents for 5 minutes.

Meanwhile, pour the vinegar into a medium pot, add the maple syrup and salt, then heat to just below the boiling point.

Once the smoking is complete, remove the smoker's lid and pour the hot vinegar mixture into the jar. Cap tightly with a regular lid. Store in a cool, dark place for 3 to 4 weeks. I like to shake the jar a once a week.

Strain and transfer the vinegar into clean bottles or similar glass containers. Store in the refrigerator or a cool, dark place (below 65°F/18°C). Shelf life for optimum flavors is around 6 months, or up to a year in perfect storage conditions.

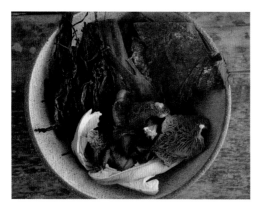

Gather your ingredients for the infusion, kelp, wood, and mushrooms here. You'll also need apple cider vinegar, maple syrup, salt, peppercorns, and 2 chili pods.

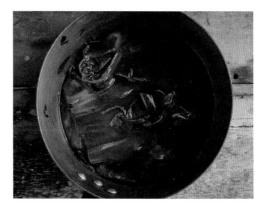

Place the part 1 ingredients in a pot and heat the contents to just below the boiling point, then let it rest for 3 to 5 minutes.

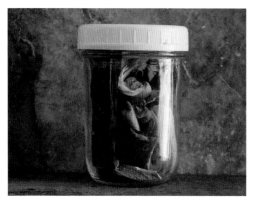

Meanwhile, for smoking, place the part 2 ingredients in a jar.

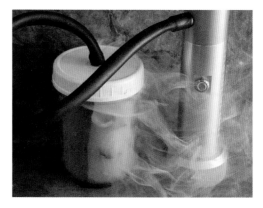

Using a handheld kitchen smoker or similar device, smoke the contents for around 5 minutes.

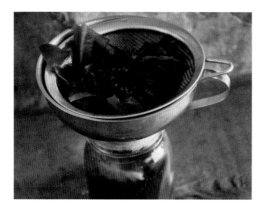

Once the smoking is complete, remove the lid and strain the original seaweed vinegar into the jar.

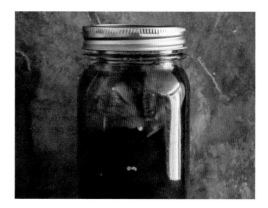

Cap tightly and place in a cool, dark place for 3 to 4 weeks, shaking occasionally. Strain, bottle, and store the final vinegar as per the instructions.

SMOKED MUSHROOMS AND
SEAWEED–INFUSED VINEGAR

This recipe is something I wanted to try for quite a while, as I love the taste of seaweed and mushrooms. I'm glad I finally did it, because the pairing is amazing. I'm sure there are different approaches to making this vinegar— this is just my method based on a few trials. I think you could simply smoke the seaweed and mushrooms together in a jar, pour in the hot vinegar, then age the contents, but this two-step method really boosts the flavors.

Ingredients for a 1-pint jar (480 ml)

1¾ cups (420 ml) apple cider vinegar
   or homemade Apple Scraps Vinegar
3 tablespoons (45 ml) maple syrup
0.35 ounces (10 g) dried kelp (kombu)
0.35 ounces (10 g) dried wakame
½ teaspoon (2.5 g) sea salt

Procedure: Part 1

Place all the ingredients in a pot and heat to just below the boiling point, then turn off the heat and let it rest for 3 to 5 minutes. Meanwhile, start part 2.

Ingredients, continued

0.5 ounces (14 g) wild oyster mushrooms,
   or you could use shiitake or other
   savory mushrooms
2 hot chili pods
0.2 ounces (5 g) dried kelp (kombu)
0.2 ounces (5 g) dried wakame
½ teaspoon (1.5 g) whole peppercorns
Wood chips for smoking, such as mesquite,
   oak, apple, hickory, and so forth
   (see Note)

Procedure: Part 2

Place all the part 2 ingredients in a pint (480 ml) jar. Use a handheld smoker to smoke the contents for 5 minutes.

Once the smoking is complete, strain the seaweed vinegar into the jar containing the smoked ingredients. Cap tightly and place in a cool, dark place for 3 to 4 weeks. I like to shake the jar a couple of times each week.

Strain and transfer the vinegar into clean bottles or similar glass containers. Seal tightly and store in the refrigerator or a cool, dark place (below 65°F/18°C). Shelf life for optimum flavors is around 6 months, or up to a year in perfect storage conditions.

Note: You can purchase handheld kitchen smokers online. You'll find them by searching for "smoke infusers," "handheld smokers," or "smoking guns." I use a brand called HANDi SMoK. Smoked wood chips such as mesquite, apple, and hickory can also be found in large supermarkets.

SMOKED HAY–INFUSED VINEGAR

Not many people know it, but cooking with hay is part of European cuisine. I remember, as a kid, tasting a leg of lamb cooked in hay. It was quite incredible. The origin of hay as a food ingredient comes from the quest to preserve food and save fuel. In the old days, the cook would bring a stew to a boil, then place the pot in a box full of hay. The insulation provided by the hay would preserve the heat and continue cooking the food for quite a while. In the process, they discovered that the hay would also flavor the food.

A modern way to cook with hay is to simply place it in the pot alongside the other ingredients. Hay can infuse some interesting sweet herbaceous flavors if you pick it at the right time.

In *Wildcrafted Fermentation*, I have a recipe for lacto-fermented ingredients in smoked hay, but while working on this book, I thought that hay could be a perfect candidate for a smoked vinegar. It takes a couple of months for optimum flavors, but it's really good in the end, with subtle "green" and smoky hints.

My wildcrafted hay-infused vinegar was mostly made of wild oats. I gather the wild oats at the end of the season (early summer in Southern California). For optimal "grassy" flavors, I collect them while they're still somewhat green and in the process of turning yellow. I don't need much—maybe 100 stalks. I simply cut the stalks at their base with scissors. Once home, I place the stalks on a table outside and let them dehydrate for a few days, then store them in a paper bag. Nothing complicated with this process. Hay can be made with all kinds of other plants, such as grasses (brome, Bermuda, and other species), wild barley (*Hordeum spontaneum*), wheat, and even legumes, such as alfalfa or clover. Just make sure that whatever you use for hay is not toxic: As a wildcrafter, you must properly identify and research any plant you intend to use. For some practical advice to get you started, see "Infusing Whole Environments," page 116.

Ingredients for a 1-quart jar (1 L)
1½ to 2 cups (20 to 25 g) "hay"

Oak, mesquite, or hickory bark chips for smoking the hay

3 cups (720 ml) raw apple cider vinegar

1½ teaspoons (7.5 g) salt

¼ cup (60 ml) maple syrup

Procedure
First, cut the hay stems (I use oat hay) in 2- to 3-inch (5 to 7.5 cm) pieces and place them in a pint (480 ml) jar. Connect the jar to a handheld kitchen smoker and smoke the contents for 4 to 5 minutes. In this recipe, I used chips from foraged oak bark, but you could also use mesquite or hickory wood chips.

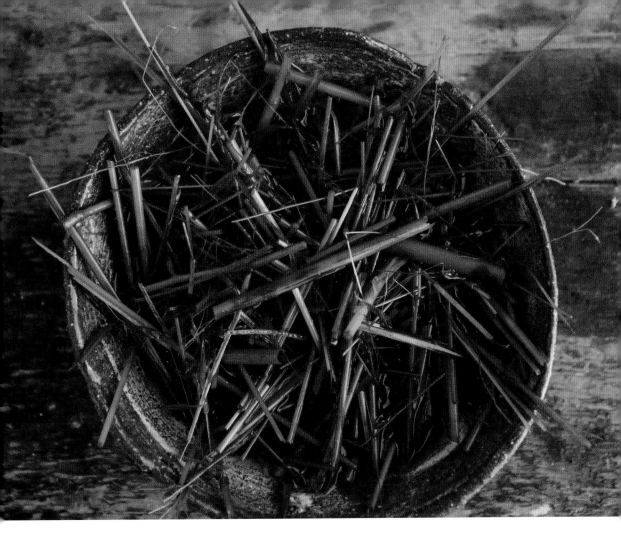

After the initial smoking is done, close the jar to let the smoke that is still inside the jar infuse the wild oats for 30 minutes.

Remove the smoked hay and place inside a quart (480 ml) jar. Add the vinegar, salt, and maple syrup. Close the jar tightly and place in a cool, dark place for at least 3 to 4 weeks. I like to shake the jar a couple of times each week. Personally, I like to wait 3 months. The end result is absolutely awesome—similar to a seasoned rice vinegar but with some interesting "hay" accents and, of course, a slight smoky touch.

Strain and transfer the vinegar into clean bottles or similar glass containers. Seal tightly and store in the refrigerator or a cool, dark place (below 65°F/18°C). Shelf life for optimum flavors is around 6 months, or up to a year in perfect storage conditions.

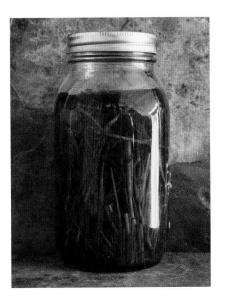

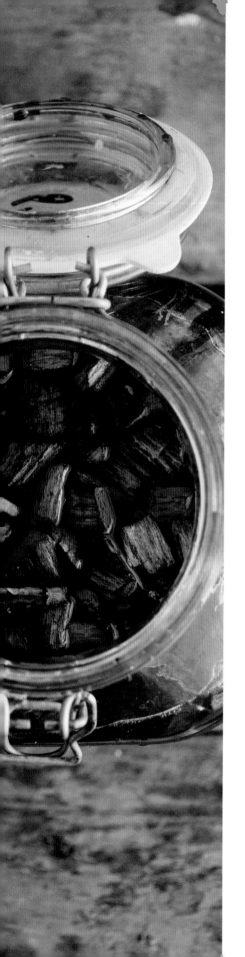

Infusing Vinegar with Wood Chips and Oak Bark

The practice of using wood to flavor fermented alcoholic beverages is quite common. It probably arose from the practice of transporting the precious liquids inside wooden barrels, from which it was discovered that specific woods added pleasant-tasting accents that enhanced the original product over time.

Nowadays, we don't need barrels to transport beer, wine, or distilled spirits, but they are still used to age beverages and imbue them with pleasing flavors. The most common wood used to make barrels is oak—usually French oak—which can add complex woody notes and hints of vanilla, hazelnuts, and clove to the stored liquid. Some barrels are also toasted, which imparts smoky flavors.

For the same reasons, barrels are also used to store and flavor vinegar. The original Orléans method, used since 1670, involves making vinegar inside oak barrels. The alcoholic beverage is placed inside a barrel laid on its side (three-quarters full). A hole is drilled at both ends of the barrel to allow for good airflow, and the liquid is left to ferment and age for several months.

Large barrels are rather inconvenient for home production, but as described in "Making Vinegar in a Barrel" (page 35), you can purchase smaller vinegar barrels ranging from 1 to 3 gallons (4 to 12 L). You're not stuck with oak; you'll find vinegar barrels made from various woods, such as acacia, ash, mulberry, cherry, pear, apple, chestnut, and more.

Unfortunately, barrels are generally rather expensive and many homebrewers resort to flavoring their boozy creations using wood cubes, chips, and spirals with various levels of toasting. Those can be purchased in homebrewing stores or online.

You don't need a huge amount of wood chips. This opens up many possibilities for wildcrafters—just make sure you thoroughly research the types of wood chips you want to collect and use. Some woods, such as yew and oleander (*Nerium oleander*), can be very toxic. As a wildcrafter, you must properly identify and research any plant you intend to use. For some practical advice to get you started, see "Infusing Whole Environments," page 116. During my travels, I have collected and used mesquite, juniper, ash, coast live oak, walnut, hickory, and olive.

I haven't experimented much with barks aside from coast live oak bark. The original idea came to me when I was foraging oak bark for a local French chef who was using it to smoke meat. I had a bunch in my storage, decided to try some in my vinegars, and loved it! I find the flavors in the bark much more complex and less tannic than the wood itself.

Foraging bark is super sustainable. I explore the forest after a good windy storm, and I always find large oak branches that have fallen on the ground. You can collect bark right then and there, but it's better to wait a few weeks for the bark to dehydrate, which makes it easier to collect.

As a note, I don't forage bark within city limits. This is particularly important if you live in a large city like Los Angeles, New York, or San Francisco. If you think about it, some city trees can be hundreds of years old, which is enough time for them to accumulate a considerable amount of dirt and pollution. In a city like Los Angeles, we're talking over 100 years of pollutant particles from car exhaust.

Aside from using bark from coast live oak, I mostly use wood chips, which I make myself using my foraging knife (made by Opinel). With a foraging knife, you can make chips from fallen branches, logs . . . whatever works.

To Toast or Not to Toast

It's not always necessary to toast wood chips for an infusion, but I always do it with vinegars. I love the smoky accents toasted wood chips provide, and I find that they can vary quite a lot based on the type of wood I use.

For strong smoky flavors, I use a kitchen torch to roast my wood chips. For a milder flavor, I place my chips in the oven on a cookie sheet and set the oven to broil. It's just a matter of supervising the process, which doesn't take long. I usually achieve a light to medium toast within 10 minutes under the broiler.

Light or medium toasting is better for bringing out woodsy flavors. A medium toast will also bring out sweetness and caramel qualities. A dark toast is typically characterized by smoky, roasty, and coffeelike flavors.

Procedure and Aging

Quantities vary based on the wood's flavors and density, but as a rough guideline, I usually use around 0.75 to 1 ounce (21 to 28 g) of toasted chips

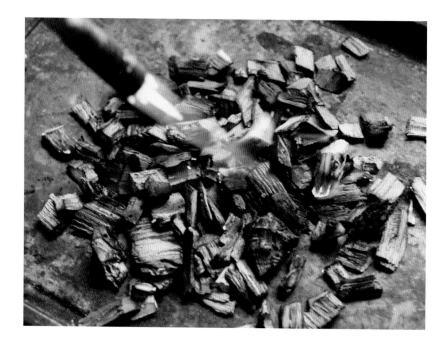

per quart (1 L) of vinegar. For roasted oak bark, 4 to 5 roasted cubes per quart (1 L), each around 1 inch (2.5 cm) wide, is a good start.

I don't heat the vinegar beforehand; I usually use a good-quality commercial apple cider vinegar or one of my homemade vinegars with at least 5 percent acidity.

Place the toasted chips in a quart (1 L) jar, add enough vinegar to fill the jar, and cap tightly. Place in a cool, dark place. Woods chips are going to float. To minimize the possibility of mold or other spoiling issues, shake or stir the contents a couple of times a day for the first 10 days. This will acidify all surfaces of the wood and reduce the risk of mold or spoiling. Age for around 6 weeks.

Strain and transfer the vinegar into clean bottles or similar glass containers. Seal tightly and store in the refrigerator or a cool, dark place (below 65°F/18°C). Shelf life for optimum flavors is around 6 months, or up to a year in perfect storage conditions.

Infusing Whole Environments

By creatively using various methods of food preservation, such as brewing, lacto-fermentation, and lacto-fermenting vinegar, you can capture the essence of entire environments. In my books I often use the word *terroir*, which comes from the French word *terre*, meaning "dirt" or "ground."

Terroir is often use in relation to wine, as in the following definition:

> The combination of factors, including soil, climate, and sunlight, that gives wine grapes their distinctive character

But terroir can also be applied to foraging and wild plants. Environments such as forests, mountains, chaparral, or deserts are endless sources of flavors unique to a specific region. A forest in Southern California has little in common with a forest in Vermont or North Carolina. Each has its specific flora and flavors.

From personal experience, even the same plants growing in different locations will taste different due to soil conditions, sunlight, altitude, and so on. In Southern California, some of the dandelions I foraged were slightly salty and tender, while in Colorado they were much more bitter and tough.

I think that diversity and uniqueness is exciting! The potential to explore a truly creative regional cuisine is wide open.

In my book *The Wildcrafting Brewer*, I explained my approach when trying to capture the flavors of a specific place. It consists of 3 steps:

1. Survey the area.
2. Establish the flavor characteristics.
3. Determine the essence of the place.

I use the same steps when researching how to create vinegars that will represent the intricacies of a whole environment at a specific moment in time (fall, spring, summer, or winter). My Mountains Vinegar is a good example of going through that process to create a hyperlocal product that is completely unique every time.

Survey the Area

The first thing I do when I want to create a vinegar that is representative of an entire landscape is simply hike the area and observe what is growing there. I usually take notes and photos while doing so. Now that I'm traveling more, I often use plant ID apps on location, then do some research and, if I have any doubts, consult with local experts to make sure the identification is correct.

Once I have the correct plant identification with its unique Latin name, then I can start doing some research as to edibility (or not), culinary history, medicinal uses, traditional methods to prepare it, potential allergies, and so on. That's one of the parts I like the most—I love doing research.

Sometimes you get real surprises. I've learned not to skip plants that seem uninteresting. For example, a couple of months ago I was exploring a location in Colorado and neglected several times to take pictures and ID a plant which, for whatever reason, I deemed a bit boring. It reminded me of a plant in Southern California that was pretty much tasteless and inedible due to its texture.

On the third morning of my daily surveying activities, I finally decided to check that plant using my ID app, not expecting anything of value. The results blew my mind. I had in front of me some American licorice, which I hadn't even known existed in the first place. The exciting part wasn't the plant; it was the roots. Since then, I've learned to pay more attention to those "boring" plants and not make assumptions.

There are no rules as to how long you need to survey an area. An experienced wildcrafter may spend a few hours, while a less-experienced person may spend days, months, or even years. My original recipe for Mountains Vinegar started with 3 ingredients. Over the years it has grown to become a blend of over 12 different ones, including berries, mushrooms, and even savory wood.

Establish the Flavor Characteristics

It will take quite a few exploration hikes to understand a place. In the beginning you may not notice all the minute details of a place and which specific berries, plants, mushrooms, and herbs grow there at various times of the year. After a while, and once you know the place well, you'll develop a sense of its base flavors.

For example, the mountain where I collect my ingredients for my Mountains Vinegar is mostly composed of pinyon pine, California juniper, and some white fir. The ratio is around 65 percent pinyon pine, 5 percent juniper, 10 percent white fir, and 20 percent various other trees such as elder, scrub oak (*Quercus ilicifolia*), black walnut, and Joshua tree (*Yucca brevifolia*) (protected). Then, to complete the picture, you have some interesting aromatic herbs such as various sages, California sagebrush, mugwort, manzanita and wild currant berries, yarrow, and many others.

I probably have 50 edible plants, berries, trees, and mushrooms (at the right time of the year) that I can collect to create something tasty. But, for an infused vinegar, you can't just take all those ingredients, stick them into a jar, pour in some vinegar, and expect something great to come out of it. This is where the art and the spiritual aspect of the flavor hunt and pairing comes to light.

Determining the Essence of the Place

The process of determining the essence of a place is a completely personal endeavor. For any given place, every single person will feel a slightly different essence because it is based on your physical and spiritual connection to the land.

My way of grasping the essence of an environment is unusual: I decide to forget everything, clear my mind, and look at the environment as if I were seeing it for the first time. It's very Zen! I just stop the constant flow of thoughts in my head, forget the list of plants I've made, and clear my mind. What is this location telling me? What do I smell and see?

It's a matter of letting the place talk to you through your senses, very much like meditation. It's a therapeutic experience in our modern, "civilized" world.

There are more components than just flavor, too. You have the aesthetics of the land, as well. While my local mountains were gorgeous, the nearby desert can be a beautifully colored place in spring but extremely harsh and dry during summer. How do you translate that aesthetic into a vinegar?

What about emotions? Do you feel uplifted or inspired by the place or do you feel sadness? Not everything has to be wonderful to create something out of it. When my favorite forest was completely burned in 2017, I made a very simple vinegar using the roasted barks from fallen oak trees, a couple of dried-up yarrow stems, and wild honey from a deserted beehive. After a few weeks of infusing, it tasted like a burnt, slightly bitter forest, which was exactly the point. I still have some of that vinegar.

What are the colors? Is it windy? A cold or warm wind? What do you smell there? Sages, pine, sagebrush?

I get a lot of my ideas and inspiration by letting an environment talk to me. You can even get a sense of the place by looking at the jar and the ingredients being infused in it.

Picking Up a Main Flavor Base

This is a little tip that can help you make elaborate concoctions. You need to start somewhere, and I think every place has one main element that could define it. For example, pinyon pine really defines the landscape in my mountain location, and I choose that as the main flavor to work from.

But there are no rules—you may have an affinity for another ingredient, such as white fir, juniper, or spruce. You could decide to go for smaller savory plants, berries, and mushrooms to interpret a landscape, too. It's all about how a place talks to you, how *you* perceive it.

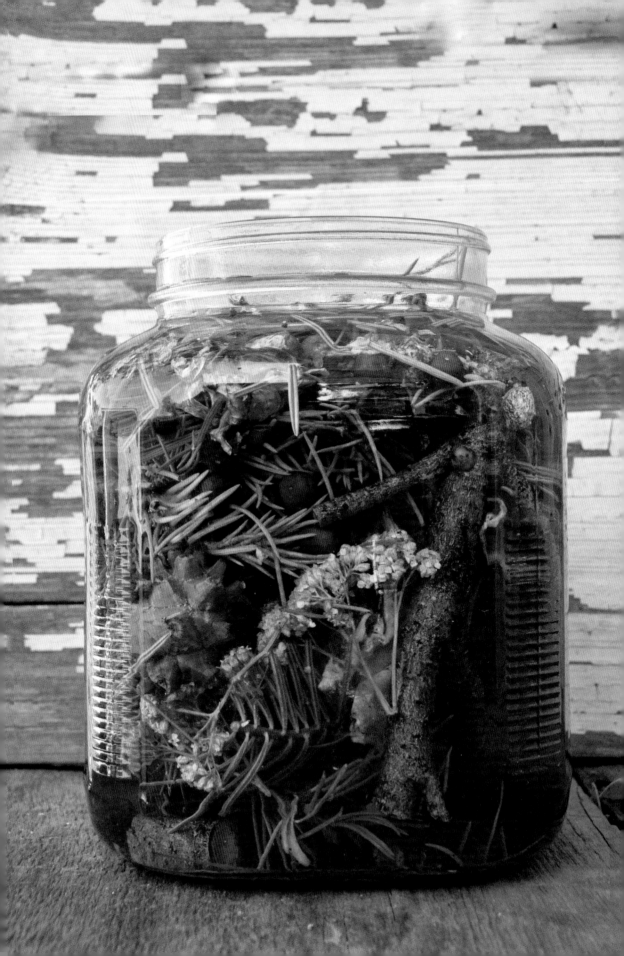

MOUNTAINS VINEGAR

This recipe is dictated by what my mountain offers at the time I visit it. I always choose mid-spring or early summer, simply because I think it's the most beautiful and plentiful time. Each year, my vinegar is different. For the last 2 years, due to a terrible local drought, it was much more austere. Climate change even plays a role.

I can give a conceptual idea of the ingredients I use (other than the vinegar), which follows the baseline ratio I mentioned earlier: 65 percent pinyon pine, 5 percent juniper berries, 10 percent white fir, and 20 percent other.

The year 2019 was a good year with decent rain, and I used the following ingredients in the following ratios:

1 gallon good-quality pasteurized
    apple cider vinegar (5 percent acidity)
Around 65 percent pinyon pine branches
    (this is my base flavor)
Around 5 percent unripe pinyon pine cones
Around 10 percent white fir
5 percent cracked green (unripe) juniper berries
    (20 berries or so)
5 percent fermented and cracked limes,
    or *loomi* (about 3 limes)

> **Note:** *The art is to understand the ratio of each plant, berry, tree, or mushroom so they pair with each other beautifully, while at the same time expressing that year's particular environment. It's a savory balancing act. For example, if you use too much mugwort, California sagebrush, or yarrow, the vinegar could end up way too bitter.*

And the following items make up the remaining 10 percent of the contents:

2 to 3 dehydrated yarrow flower heads
5 to 6 dehydrated mugwort leaves
20 to 30 manzanita berries
1 sprig California sagebrush
4 turkey tail mushrooms
Dried elderberries

Infusing and Aging the Vinegar

Unlike many of the infused vinegars in this book, this Mountains Vinegar can be aged for a long time. Pine, fir, and spruce seem to benefit from longer aging, but it's up to your personal preference.

The reason I use a pasteurized vinegar for this one is due to that extreme aging. I age the infused vinegar for 2 to 6 months at room temperature. I'm breaking a lot of rules related to vinegar infusion methods, but the end product is totally food safe (it has a low pH) and incredibly delicious—hints of pine and tangerine, sweet and bitter at the same time, a touch of cinnamon. I always say it tastes a bit like Christmas.

By the way, it's not unusual for a mother of vinegar to form on top even if the original vinegar was pasteurized. This is probably because a mild alcoholic fermentation occurs due to the presence of wild yeast, followed by acetic acid fermentation by the *Acetobacter* present on the ingredients.

Flavor Profiles

Pinyon pine tastes like sweet candy with tangerine, orange, lemon, and pine hints. The strongest flavor is inside the branches, which I crack or cut into small 1-inch (2.5 cm) pieces.

White fir has strong tangerine and lemony flavors.

California juniper berries taste like pine when green. When they are blue and ripe, they are extremely sweet but not as flavorful.

Yarrow, **California sagebrush**, and **mugwort** are highly aromatic plants, a bit hoppy and bitter.

Manzanita tastes like sweet apples.

Turkey tail mushrooms contributed some earthy, mushroomy flavors when fresh. They can be bitter if boiled.

Elderberries have an interesting fruity accent, but they are not too sweet. They're kind of earthy and tart, too.

Fermented limes (or loomi) have an amazing, complex tart and sour pungency that pairs beautifully with pine and fir. They are not part of the mountain environment, but they make such a wonderful contribution to the overall flavor profile that I now use them in my Mountains Vinegars. They're dehydrated limes, but the dehydration process is long enough that they ferment inside, which gives them a wonderful savory punch. You can search online for "loomi limes" if you want more information about the process for making them.

Once the initial infusion is done, strain and transfer the vinegar into clean bottles or similar glass containers. Seal tightly and store in the refrigerator or a cool, dark place. This will taste awesome for years.

It's one of my favorite vinegars for making shrubs (vinegar drinks), but I also use it for salad dressings, canning, and lots of quick pickles.

What can you create with your local mountain, forest, chaparral, or desert?

CHAPTER 4

Wilder Vinaigrettes, Salad Dressings, and Sauces

During springtime, one of the easiest ways to use fresh wild greens is to make a salad. Southern California was a paradise in terms of providing me ways to create delicious wild food salads that truly represented nature's bounty. We're talking purslane (*Portulaca oleracea*), dandelion, wild fennel, chickweed, wild chervil, mustard and radish sprouts, wood sorrel (*Oxalis* spp.), miner's lettuce, wild onions, and so on. But, with some experience or by mixing regular and wild greens, I think it's possible to create something delicious wherever you live, unless you're located in the artic or desert.

Making a great wild food salad is an art form, and you can bring it to the next level by using your homemade vinegar to create delicious vinaigrettes or salad dressings.

To eliminate any confusion, a vinaigrette is a type of dressing that is usually simpler and lighter than those that incorporate creamy ingredients such as yogurt, cream, peanut butter, and so on. Vinaigrettes are typically a tasty combination of oil, vinegar, savory herbs, and spices.

That said, I thought I should write about seasoned vinegars first, as I use them for most of my sauces and vinaigrette recipes.

Before I started making my own vinegar, seasoned rice vinegar was my favorite. Not only was it delicious, but it was extremely versatile. I used it to make a lot of the quick pickles I served at my foraging classes.

Quick pickles, in case you're not familiar with them, are also known as refrigerator pickles. They're simply ingredients that are pickled in a solution composed of vinegar, water, salt, and sometimes sugar, then stored in the refrigerator for a somewhat short period of time ranging from a few days to weeks. (You'll find more information about quick pickles in chapter 6).

Although rice vinegar is quite flavorless compared to other commercial vinegars, such as red wine vinegar or balsamic vinegar, it always seemed to boost the flavors of my ingredients. I knew that seasoned rice vinegar was made from the rice brewed to make sake, but I figured there must be something quite esoteric about the process.

When I started to make my own vinegars and experiment with them, I decided to look at how seasoned rice vinegar was made. To my utter surprise, the secret was just the addition of sugar and salt in perfect balance. The recipe for seasoned rice vinegar is extremely simple:

> 1 cup (240 ml) rice vinegar
> ¼ cup (50 g) regular white sugar
> 2 teaspoons (10 g) salt

Mix and stir all the ingredients together until the sugar is dissolved, and voila! You're done.

Before I encountered this recipe, I made most of my quick pickles with pure vinegars and maybe a bit of salt. Learning to season my (wilder) homemade vinegars really brought my quick pickles and canning recipes to a new level. The only change I've made in recent years is to reduce the amount of white sugar I use and replace it with more organic ingredients such as maple syrup or honey.

My usual recipe is:

> ¼ cup (60 ml) homemade vinegar
> 2 teaspoons (10 ml) maple syrup or honey
> ½ teaspoon (2.5 g) salt

So, for 1 cup (240 ml) of vinegar, you're looking at:

> 2½ tablespoons (37 ml) maple syrup or honey
> 2 teaspoons (10 g) salt

The seasoning is quite delicious with homemade or commercial apple cider vinegar, but it truly shines with more unusual and complex vinegars such as Elderberry Wine Vinegar or Mugwort Beer Vinegar. When I make my quick pickles, I often dilute the vinegar with water so it complements rather than competes with the flavorful ingredients. My basic quick pickle vinegar recipe goes something like this:

> 3 tablespoons (45 ml) vinegar
> 3 tablespoons (45 ml) water
> 2 teaspoons (10 ml) maple syrup or honey
> ½ teaspoon (2.5 g) salt

Of course, you can add more vinegar, pickling or other spices, savory herbs, and the like.

SLICED CATTAIL SHOOT QUICK PICKLE

Here is a good example of using a homemade seasoned vinegar. It's a simple quick pickle I made for one of my classes.

Cattail (*Typha latifolia*) can be found throughout the Northern Hemisphere. The plant loves water and grows in streams and wetland habitats. It's usually 5 to 8 feet (1.5 to 2.4 m) tall once mature. It is easily recognizable with its stiff, flat leaf blades. In the center you will find an erect, rounded stem reaching up to 6 to 7 feet (1.8 to 2.1 m) in height. At the tip of the stem, the flower head forms a characteristic brown cylinder.

You want to forage cattail before it flowers, when the shoot is still very tender. The plant is usually 4 to 5 feet (1.2 to 1.5 m) tall at that stage. The bottom of the stem looks quite similar to a leek. To extract the shoot, my method is to push aside the largest two leaves, grab the inner part of the stem close to the ground or water, and pull gently. It should come up easily. Remove the top part (green leaves), as you're mostly interested in the lower tender part.

Once home, thoroughly clean the collected shoots in cold water. Slice horizontally and remove the outside layers if they are a bit too tough or stringy, then vertically slice the tender shoot.

Ingredients for a ½-pint jar (240 ml)

- 2 tablespoons (30 ml) Mugwort Beer Vinegar (or apple cider vinegar)
- 1½ teaspoons (7.5 ml) maple syrup or honey
- ⅓ teaspoon (1.6 g) salt
- 4 ounces (120 g) sliced cattail shoots
- 1 tablespoon (3.5 g) chopped wild chervil (or substitute dill or parsley— dill is much better!)
- 2 tablespoons (30 ml) water

Procedure

Mix the vinegar with the maple syrup and salt. Stir until the syrup or honey is dissolved properly.

Fill a ½-pint (240 ml) jar with sliced cattail shoots, then add the chervil, water, and seasoned vinegar.

As a quick pickle, I think cattail is much better if aged overnight and consumed within 2 to 3 days. If you age it too long it becomes a bit mushy, probably due to the high starch content.

Drain the brine before serving.

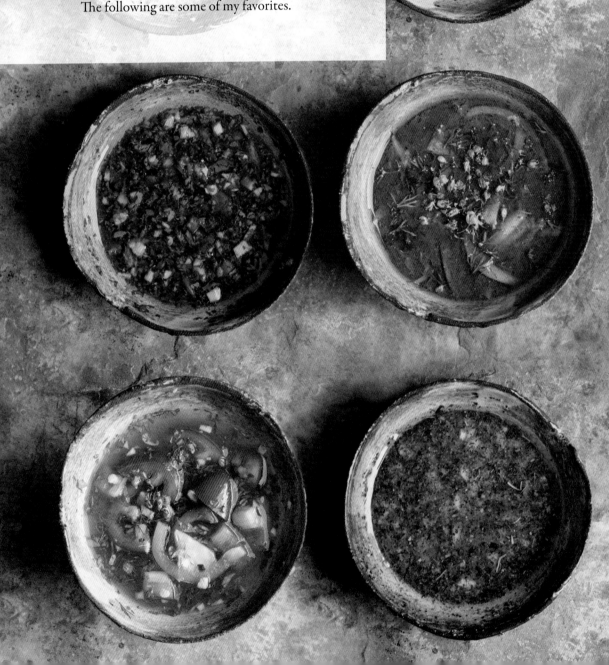

Vinaigrette and Salad Dressing Recipes

A lot of classic recipes can be adapted to include your homemade vinegar and ingredients found in your environment. When you use what nature provides, you have the opportunity to create truly unique vinaigrettes and dressings.

The following are some of my favorites.

SPICY FOREST GREENS
SALAD DRESSING

This is the perfect dressing for exploring your local terroir. The number of possible experimentations is mind-boggling. You can make this recipe using all kinds of wild greens, such as dandelion, young nettles, various wild mustard leaves, curly dock, watercress, wild mints, purslane, sweet white clover, wild onions, garlic mustard, chervil, miner's lettuce, winter cress (*Barbarea vulgaris*), chickweed, and so on.

The art is to use wild herbs that will blend with and complement each other beautifully. Don't be afraid to experiment and learn from your failures. In no time you'll be able to create some delicious vinaigrettes.

My personal favorite greens blend in Southern California is as follows:

¼ cup (7 g) chickweed
¼ cup (7 g) wild chervil (you can use parsley)
¼ cup (7 g) miner's lettuce

To this, I could add flavor accents such as a bit of sweet white clover, watercress, young curly dock leaves, or wood sorrel (lemony).

If you are using commercial savory herbs, you can experiment with basic herbs such as parsley, chervil, arugula, Italian parsley, carrot greens, celery leaves, and cilantro. For strong accents you could use basil, thyme, chives, tarragon, and the like.

My favorite vinegar for this vinaigrette is my Mountains Vinegar, but a seasoned homemade apple cider vinegar also works very well.

Ingredients for a ½-pint jar (240 ml)—three-quarters full

¾ to 1 cup (21 to 28 g) mixed forest (or commercial) greens, loosely packed
6 tablespoons (90 ml) Mountains Vinegar or seasoned apple cider vinegar
Juice of one lemon
2 tablespoons (30 ml) olive or avocado oil
1 medium jalapeño pepper, minced
2 teaspoons (6 g) minced onion
1 garlic clove, minced

Procedure

Mix all the ingredients together in a bowl. Transfer into a pint (240 ml) jar, secure the lid, and shake vigorously for a few seconds.

Store in the fridge for at least a couple of hours before serving. This will allow the flavors to blend together.

THAI-INSPIRED VINAIGRETTE

I love Thai food and I love spice. This recipe is definitely on the spicy side. You can substitute the Thai chili peppers with milder ones, such as jalapeños or serrano peppers; or if you like pain, you can use habanero or Scotch bonnet peppers instead. Thai peppers pack the heat, and they are measured at 50,000 to 100,000 Scoville heat units. On the Scoville scale, that's just below habaneros, which are measured between 100,000 to 350,000 heat units. For more on the Scoville heat units, see "How Spicy Is It?" on page 162.

I use a lot of nontraditional Thai ingredients, which is why I don't pretend I'm making a Thai vinaigrette. It's hard to beat the flavor of fish sauce, but if your diet is plant-based you can substitute it with soy sauce or Bragg Liquid Aminos.

On the wilder side, feel free to substitute the cilantro with chervil (wild or commercial), chickweed, watercress, or a mix of wildcrafted savory herbs.

It's hard to beat a good homemade apple cider vinegar with this recipe, but I've also made it using Mugwort Beer Vinegar or white wine vinegar with success.

This vinaigrette can also be used as a dipping sauce.

Ingredients for a
½-pint jar (240 ml)

3 tablespoons (45 ml) lime juice

3 tablespoons (5 g) roughly minced cilantro
   or wild greens

2 tablespoons (30 ml) raw apple cider vinegar

2 tablespoons (30 ml) water

1 tablespoon (15 ml) maple syrup, honey,
   or sugar

2 teaspoons (10 ml) fish sauce or soy sauce

2 teaspoons (6 g) minced red onion

1 to 2 teaspoons (1.5 to 3 g)
   thinly sliced Thai chili peppers

1 teaspoon (3 g) minced garlic

1 teaspoon (2 g) grated fresh ginger

Procedure

Mix all the ingredients together in a bowl. Transfer into the jar, secure the lid, and shake vigorously for a few seconds.

Store in the fridge for at least a couple of hours before serving. This will allow the flavors to blend. It should keep in the fridge for at least a week, but it's much better fresh. If you want to store the vinaigrette for a while, it's better to skip the minced cilantro to start or wild greens and add them a couple of hours before serving. Old cilantro and many wild greens will not look fantastic after marinating for a couple of days in an acidic liquid.

BLACK MUSTARD POWDER VINAIGRETTE

There are around 40 different species of mustard plant, but not all of them will work for this recipe. You're pretty much stuck foraging black mustard seeds, if you are a wildcrafter, or purchasing store-bought mustard powder, which uses white/yellow mustard (*Sinapis alba*) or brown mustard (*Brassica juncea*). In Los Angeles I found a local grocery store specializing in foods from the Middle East, which sold black mustard seeds, but I've not been able to find them anywhere else.

If you are using black mustard seeds, be aware that inhaling the powder can cause severe airway irritation (similar to black pepper).

Freshly ground black mustard seeds will taste bitter for the first 2 to 3 days, but then the bitterness goes away. Take this into account when you prepare the vinaigrette.

As with Thai-Inspired Vinaigrette, this makes a terrific dipping sauce, as well.

Ingredients for a ¼-pint jar (120 ml)

3 tablespoons (45 ml) raw apple cider vinegar (see Note)
2 tablespoons (30 ml) soy sauce
1 tablespoon (15 ml) water
1 tablespoon (9 g) black mustard seeds or store-bought mustard powder
1 teaspoon (5 ml) sesame oil
1 teaspoon (5 ml) maple syrup or honey
1 teaspoon (3 g) onion powder
1 teaspoon (3 g) chili flakes (optional)

Note: This recipe also works well with prickly pear vinegar, red wine vinegar, and white wine vinegar.

Procedure

If you are using wildcrafted black mustard seeds, make a powder using a *molcajete* (Mexican stone grinder) or electric coffee grinder.

Mix all the ingredients together in a bowl, then transfer them into the jar and shake well. Store in the fridge for at least 3 days before serving. If you use black mustard seeds, storing in the refrigerator will reduce the bitterness. It's not an issue with store-bought mustard powder.

Black mustard is considered invasive in some parts of Los Angeles. This is a good example of how a plant that is grown as a crop in different countries is demonized and completely unused in the United States. Many undesirable plants can be turned into gourmet food, which frankly is so much better than trying to eradicate them using herbicides!

WILDER CURRY VINAIGRETTE

I think this vinaigrette goes well with wild food salads that have a bit of a bitter edge. For example, salads with a decent amount of dandelion, arugula, or similar bitter greens. That said, it works nicely with milder salads, too.

There aren't many wild ingredients aside from the vinegar itself in the basic recipe, but adding a small amount of savory wild or store-bought herbs such as dill, wild fennel, desert parsley (*Lomatium foeniculaceum*), watercress, or parsley can do wonders. In a recent recipe version, I added ½ teaspoon (0.2 g) of fresh dill (a weed in Colorado) and sprinkled in some of the dehydrated wild onion flowers I found in the mountains.

This was quite delicious and complex with my Mountains Vinegar and Pine-, Fir-, and Spruce-Infused Vinegars, but this vinaigrette is so tasty that a simple apple cider vinegar will also work.

Ingredients for a ¼-pint jar (120 ml)

3 tablespoons (45 ml) Mountains Vinegar or homemade raw apple cider vinegar

2 tablespoons (30 ml) olive or avocado oil

1 tablespoon (15 ml) lemon juice

2 teaspoons (10 ml) maple syrup

0.3 ounce (8 g) sliced red onions

1 teaspoon (3 g) curry powder

½ teaspoon (2.5 g) salt

½ teaspoon (1.5 g) garlic powder

½ teaspoon (1.5 g) powdered savory wild herbs (fennel, dill, or others)

Procedure

Mix all the ingredients together in a bowl, then transfer into the jar, secure the lid, and shake vigorously for a few seconds.

Store in the fridge for at least a couple of hours before serving. This will allow the flavors to blend together. It should keep in the fridge for at least a week, but it's much better fresh (within 48 hours).

CHUNKY JALAPEÑO VINAIGRETTE

This dressing is somewhat thick—sort of a mix between a salsa and a vinaigrette. Personally, I keep the jalapeño quite chunky and thus crunchy. I've used this dressing for wild food salads featuring wild edibles that are on the bland side, such as sow thistle (*Sonchus* spp.), dandelion, mallow, cattail, and so on.

Taste the jalapeño first, as some of them can be quite spicy. You can make the same recipe using bell pepper as a base if you want. The added wild greens in this recipe should pack a punch—we're talking wild fennel, dill weed (*Anethum graveolens*), chervil, or chickweed. Some mints, such as water mint, would work nicely, too. You can make a mix of them.

Instead of wild greens, you can also use store-bought parsley, chervil, dill, oregano, basil, or dried herb blends such as herbes de Provence or Italian herbs.

Ingredients for a ¼-pint jar (120 ml)

¼ cup (60 ml) unpasteurized
   apple cider vinegar
1 large jalapeño (spicy or not),
   chopped in large chunks
1 garlic clove, minced
1 tablespoon (9 g) chopped red onion
1 tablespoon (4 g) minced savory wild
   greens (fennel, dill, chickweed, chervil)
2 teaspoons (10 ml) maple syrup
1 teaspoon (2 g) freshly grated ginger
½ teaspoon (2.5 g) salt

Procedure

Mix all the ingredients together in a bowl, then transfer into a jar. Shake vigorously for a few seconds.

Store in the fridge for at least a couple of hours before serving. This will allow the flavors to blend together. It should keep in the fridge for at least a week, but it's much better fresh (within 48 hours).

If you want to store the vinaigrette for a while, it's better to skip the wild greens to start and add them a couple of hours before serving. Many wild greens will not look fantastic after marinating for a couple of days in an acidic liquid. If you use dried herbs rather than fresh wild herbs, this won't be an issue.

WILD DIJON VINAIGRETTE

This is a classic vinaigrette made wilder. In fact, it's completely wild and a good example of creating a tasty vinaigrette with ingredients sourced from nature. You can't find flavors like this in mass-market products. For this recipe, I use my Stone-Ground Wild Black Mustard made with black mustard seeds, salt that I sourced from Oregon seawater, and olive oil from local "feral" olives. You can create a similar vinaigrette with organic store-bought ingredients.

Ingredients for a ¼-pint jar (120 ml)

¼ cup (60 ml) Apple Scraps Vinegar, Mugwort Beer Vinegar, or Mountains Vinegar

2½ tablespoons (37 ml) stone-ground black mustard or store-bought Dijon mustard

½ teaspoon (2.5 g) salt

1 tablespoon (15 ml) maple syrup

⅓ cup (80 ml) olive oil

Procedure

In a bowl, mix together the vinegar, mustard, salt, and maple syrup, then gradually whisk in the olive oil. It's much better when served right away, but you can also make enough to bottle and store in the fridge. You'll need to shake or whisk before serving.

You can easily store this vinaigrette in the fridge for at least 3 months.

A wild food salad made with chickweed, shredded dandelion, fermented and quick-pickled wild radish pods and burdock root, black mustard sprouts, carrots, Korean radish, wild watercress, and pickled "feral" olives with my Wild Dijon Vinaigrette.

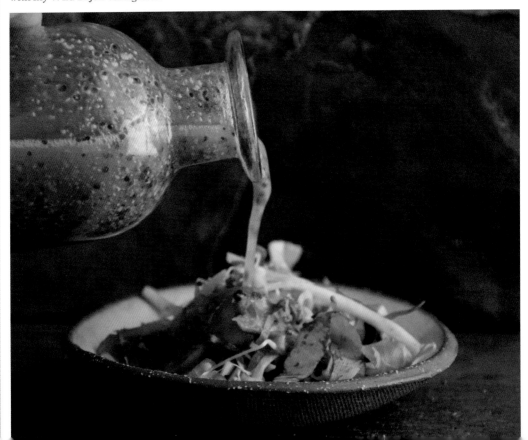

FOREST HERBS VINEGARY PASTE

I always try to find ways to preserve my favorite wild greens and their incredible flavors through different traditional methods, such as dehydration, fermentation, and so on. Making vinegar is another delicious option.

I thought that the idea of preserving herb pastes in vinegar was quite common and that such a product could even be purchased at the store, but the only version I found contained ascorbic acid and citric acid as preservatives as well as other unusual ingredients like whey, glycerin, xanthan gum, dextrose, and so on. I tried a couple, and I was less than impressed with the flavor and texture.

You can find somewhat similar condiments—for example, traditional British or French "green sauces" or salsa verde in the United States and South America.

I keep the recipe super simple. This kind of paste can be made with many different tasty wild greens, including watercress, garlic mustard (*Alliaria petiolata*), nettles, curly dock, wild arugula, knotweed, and wood sorrel. I've prepared this recipe with store-bought parsley and dried Italian herbs, and it tasted fantastic.

You can add grated fresh ginger if you want—I made it optional because my chosen wild herbs have a lot of flavors already (chickweed or chervil) and I like to focus on those.

Ingredients for a ¼-pint jar (120 ml)

4 ounces (120 g) coarsely chopped
  forest herbs (chickweed, chervil,
  miner's lettuce, or others)
¼ cup (60 ml) seasoned rice vinegar
  or apple cider vinegar
½ medium red onion, minced
2 garlic cloves, coarsely chopped
1 teaspoon (2 g) grated fresh ginger
  (optional)
¼ teaspoon (0.8 g) ground peppercorns

Procedure

Place all your ingredients into a mortar or food processor and make a rough paste.

Transfer the paste into a small jar, close the top, and store in the fridge. It will keep for a long time; I'm still using the forest paste I made 4 months ago.

I use this paste as a flavorful additive to sandwiches, vegan burritos, creative amuse-bouches, and even soups. You can also serve it with sliced roast meat, and it's quite good on fish, too.

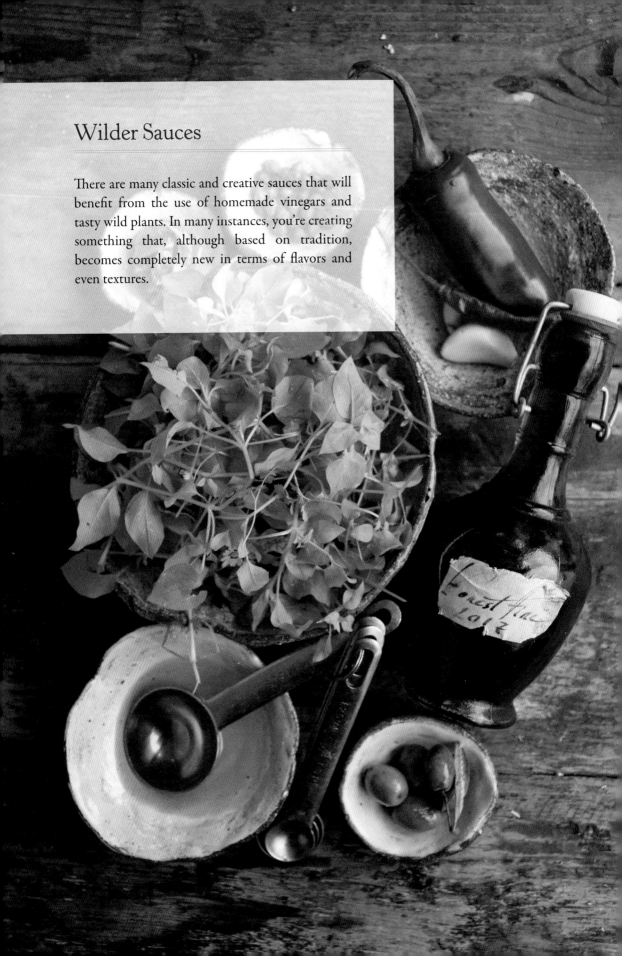

Wilder Sauces

There are many classic and creative sauces that will benefit from the use of homemade vinegars and tasty wild plants. In many instances, you're creating something that, although based on tradition, becomes completely new in terms of flavors and even textures.

WASABI GINGER VINEGAR SAUCE

This sauce works very well with seafood (sashimi, oysters, mussels, clams), but I also use it when I make a sashimi with fermented oyster mushrooms. It's also very good with sliced cucumber and a sprinkle of dill or fennel.

This sauce is quite spicy, but you can tone down the heat if you want by reducing the amount of wasabi paste.

Ingredients for slightly more than ¼ cup (60 ml)

2 tablespoons (30 ml) olive oil

2 tablespoons (30 ml) unpasteurized apple cider vinegar or white wine vinegar

2 teaspoons (12 g) wasabi paste (see Note)

1½ teaspoons (7 ml) maple syrup, honey, or palm sugar

1 teaspoon (4 g) grated fresh ginger

1 teaspoon (2 g) minced chickweed, wild chervil, dill, parsley, or similar savory plant

½ teaspoon (5 g) salt

Procedure

Combine the ingredients in a small bowl and mix everything together. Wait a few minutes for the flavors to blend before using it.

If you want to make the sauce thinner and more fluid, grind the minced chickweed, salt, and grated ginger into a thin paste with a grinder or mortar and pestle, then add the oil, vinegar, maple syrup, and wasabi paste. Grind a few more minutes, then strain.

The sauce can be stored in the fridge for a week or so.

Note: No wasabi at home? You can substitute the wasabi paste with 1 tablespoon of Stone-Ground Wild Black Mustard or store-bought Dijon mustard. It's not as awesome as the wasabi, but hey . . . it will work!

ELDERBERRY SOY VINEGAR SAUCE

This is another sauce I've used with a fermented oyster mushroom sashimi. It is similar to some ponzu sauce recipes, but I don't want to call it a ponzu sauce due to the wild ingredients used.

Ingredients for about ¼ pint jar (120 ml)

- 2 teaspoons (5 g) dried elderberries (optional), see Note
- ¼ cup (60 ml) smoked seaweed vinegar (or rice vinegar), more if needed
- 3 tablespoons plus 1 teaspoon (50 ml) soy sauce
- 2 tablespoons (30 ml) orange juice
- 2 tablespoons (30 ml) elderberry wine or regular red wine (see Note)
- 1 tablespoon (15 ml) lime juice
- 1 teaspoon (5 ml) maple syrup
- 1 teaspoon (1.5 g) grated orange zest (optional)
- ¼ teaspoon (0.5 g) chili flakes

Procedure

If you are using dried elderberries, combine them with the vinegar and bring the solution to a simmer for 3 to 4 minutes. Use a bit more than ¼ cup (60 ml) of vinegar to account for evaporation. Let it cool off slowly. If you are omitting the elderberries, begin with the next step.

Place all the ingredients in a jar, close the lid, and shake. Place the jar in the fridge overnight and strain before serving. It will keep for up to a month.

> *Note:* I really like the combination of soy sauce and elderberries, but I understand that elderberries are not something you can source easily (although it's possible to buy the berries and wine online). You can substitute the elderberry wine with regular red wine or mirin (a sweet Japanese cooking wine).

BARBECUE SAUCE

If you make a book about vinegars, you can't escape having to include a recipe for barbecue sauce. It's one of the oldest sauces in North America, with roots in European, Native American, and African cultures. A good barbecue sauce is the perfect balance of sweet, sour, spicy, and salty. And from that base you can add flavors such as garlic, curry, liquid smoke, spices and aromatic herbs, onion, and so on.

While barbecue sauce is mostly associated with pork, it's also fantastic with chicken and fish (including shellfish). If your diet is plant-based, I think a good barbecue sauce is awesome with mushrooms, too.

My favorite barbecue sauce recipe with non-foraged ingredients is as follows.

Ingredients for a 1-pint jar (480 ml)

1½ cups (360) apple cider vinegar
    or homemade Apple Scraps Vinegar
¼ cup (60 ml) tomato sauce (canned)
2 tablespoons (30 ml) molasses
1 to 2 teaspoons (2 to 4 g) chili flakes
    (mild or spicy)
1 teaspoon (3 g) ground black pepper
1 teaspoon (5 g) salt
1 teaspoon (3 g) onion powder
1 teaspoon (3 g) garlic powder
½ teaspoon (2.5 ml) liquid smoke
½ teaspoon (1.5 g) paprika powder
½ teaspoon (1.5 g) curry powder

Procedure

Combine all the ingredients in a bowl and whisk together. Transfer to a saucepan over medium heat and bring to a slow simmer.

Simmer for at least 5 minutes or to the consistency you like.

You can serve the sauce right away, or transfer it to a pint jar, seal, and store in the fridge. It should last for at least a month.

SOUTHERN CALIFORNIA
BARBECUE SAUCE

Now that we've done a regular barbecue sauce, let's create one that incorporates local flavors.

Most people don't realize it, but you can definitely take a basic barbecue sauce recipe and transform it into a unique local delicacy through the use of a good homemade vinegar made from fermented local berries or fruits, as well as the addition of local herbs and spices.

The vast majority of barbecue sauces will ask for apple cider vinegar, while a few recommend red or white wine vinegar. However, I like to use a strong and bold vinegar as a base, such as Elderberry Wine or Blackberry Wine Vinegar.

Infused vinegars are also perfect. For example, in this recipe I use a blend of elderberry and red wine vinegars infused with roasted oak bark. This makes the final sauce taste like it has been aged in a toasted oak barrel.

This recipe is particular to Southern California, as it uses a wild spice blend of local sages, California sagebrush, and bay leaves.

Ingredients

1 cup (240 ml) blended red wine vinegar and Elderberry Wine Vinegar, infused with local roasted oak bark

6 tablespoons (90 ml) tomato sauce (canned or homemade)

2 tablespoons (30 ml) molasses or maple syrup

1 tablespoon (6 g) Southern California Wild Spice Blend

2 teaspoons (4 g) chili flakes (spicy or not)

1 teaspoon (3 g) paprika

1 teaspoon (3 g) onion powder

½ teaspoon (2.5 ml) liquid smoke

Procedure

Combine all the ingredients in a bowl and whisk together. Transfer to a saucepan over medium heat and bring to a slow simmer.

Simmer for at least 5 minutes or to the consistency you like.

You can serve the sauce right away or transfer it to a pint jar, seal, and store in the fridge. It should last for at least a month.

Southern California Wild Spice Blend

The ingredients for my Southern California spice blend are as follows.
You'll need to set your scale to grams for this.

Ingredients

4 grams white sage
2 grams California sagebrush
5 grams black sage
32 grams garlic powder
25 grams coarse salt
1 gram California bay leaf
6 grams whole peppercorns

Procedure

Reduce the ingredients to a crude powder using an electric or stone grinder.

Immediately place in a jar, seal, and wait a couple of days before using so the flavors can blend. If stored in a cool, dark place, this spice blend will last for at least a year. This spice blend packs *a lot* of flavor—no need to use a huge amount.

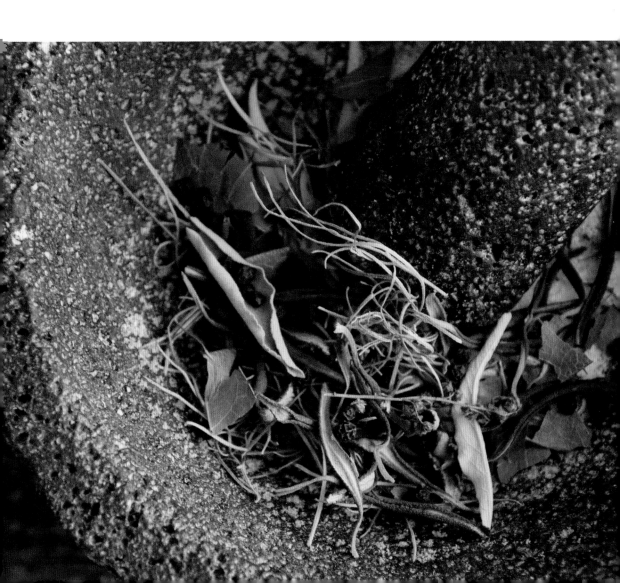

BLUEBERRIES AIGRE-DOUX

This is a traditional sauce recipe from Belgium and France that we used to make with local blackberries, but it works perfectly with any kind of berry. I've even made one with prickly pears. Traditionally, this kind of sauce was mostly served with game meat, such as pheasant, quail, or rabbit, but I think it works nicely with mushrooms. It was quite delicious with the plant-based acorn burgers I made a couple of years ago.

Aigre-doux is French for "sour and sweet." Vinegar is the base for sourness and, in this case, maple syrup is for sweetness. But you can also use regular sugar or honey.

For this aigre-doux I use elderberry wine and Elderberry Wine Vinegar. Try it with a dish that features roasted oyster mushrooms—the flavor combination of elderberries with the earthiness of mushrooms is fantastic.

Of course, you can use commercial red wine vinegar and red wine. The sauce is sublime with wildcrafted blueberries—realize that some store-bought blueberries can be completely tasteless.

Ingredients for three ½-pint jars (240 ml)

2 cups (380 g) blueberries

1½ cups (360 ml) elderberry wine
  (or regular red wine)

½ cup (120 ml) Elderberry Wine Vinegar
  (or red wine vinegar)

¼ cup (60 ml) maple syrup
  (or honey or white sugar)

Juice of 1 lemon

2 to 3 teaspoons (4 to 6 g) grated ginger

Procedure

Place everything except the ginger into a saucepan or pot. Bring to a boil, then a slow simmer, and reduce the sauce for around 15 minutes. No real rules—I like it quite thick. The ginger is traditionally added in the last 3 to 4 minutes of simmering.

Transfer to a jar and place in the fridge, where it will keep for at least 2 weeks.

This blueberries aigre-doux recipe is a good base, but you can expand it creatively. I think adding clove or cinnamon could do wonders. I added a few California sagebrush stems as flavoring in the jar on the facing page.

So, there you go—something to try with all kinds of wild berries or even fruits.

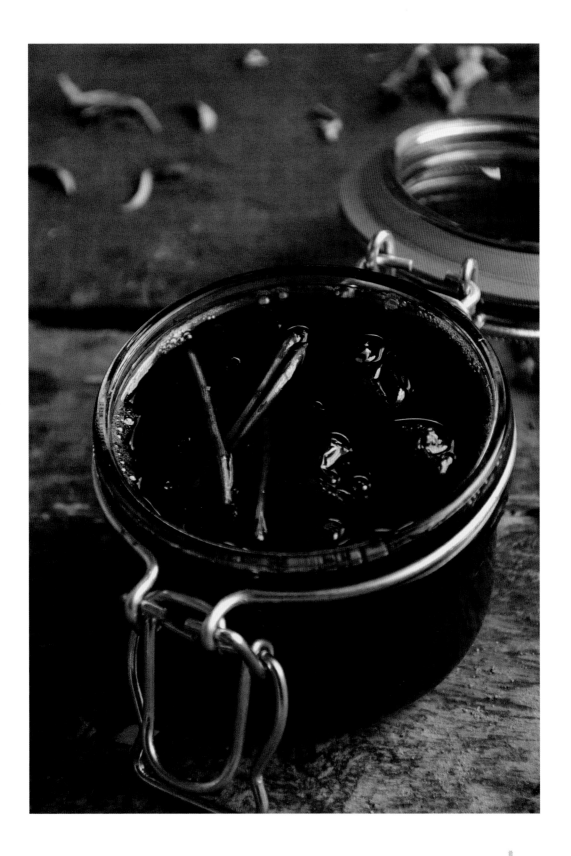

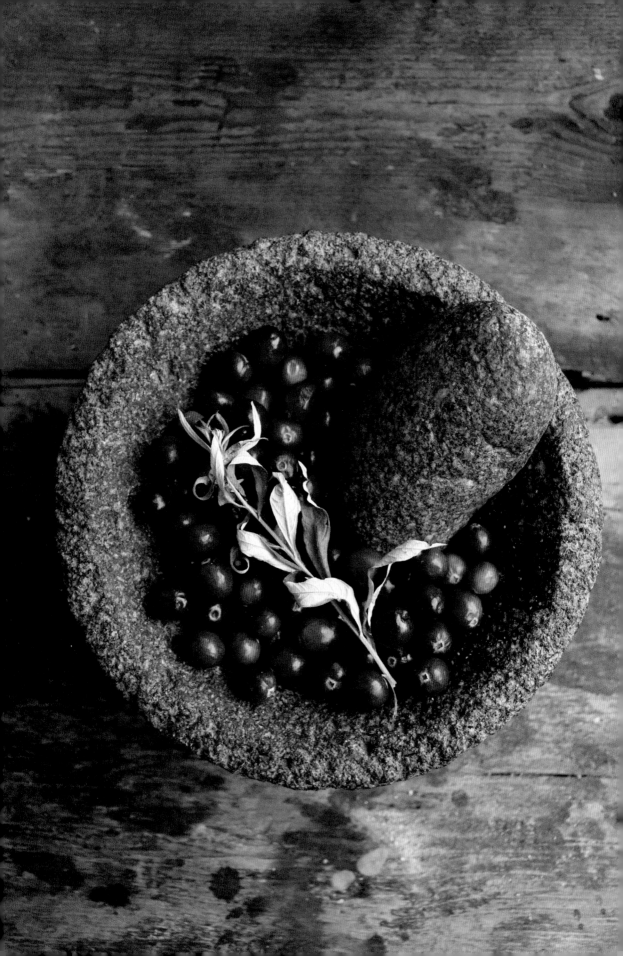

RAW CRANBERRY VINEGAR SAUCE/JAM

Normally I'm not a fan of cranberry, but this sauce is quite awesome and so simple to make. You can think of it as a jam, too. The key is a great-tasting homemade vinegar, but you can also pick up some good-quality commercial apple cider vinegar (like Bragg).

The recipe is adaptable to a lot of wild or commercial berries. You can skip the mugwort if you want. There are many other awesome herbs to pair with cranberries, such as culinary sage, thyme, water mint, ginger, cinnamon, cloves, and the like. But, being a wildcrafter, I like to add a touch of my own terroir.

This is a raw recipe, so you get some probiotics from the raw vinegar.

Ingredients

5 ounces (140 g) cranberries
3 to 4 tablespoons (45 to 60 ml)
   raw apple cider vinegar
3 tablespoons (45 ml) maple syrup (or honey)
Pinch of salt
Pinch of chili flakes (optional)
2 mugwort leaves or herb of your choice
2 teaspoons (7 g) chia seeds
   (*Salvia columbariae*)

Procedure

Place everything but the mugwort and chia in a blender (or stone grinder). Blend to the consistency of your liking. When done, transfer to a pint jar, add the chia seeds and mugwort leaves, then stir.

It is best to age the sauce for 3 to 4 days in the fridge before serving so the mugwort can do its magic. Remove the leaves before serving.

This will easily keep in the fridge for a couple of weeks.

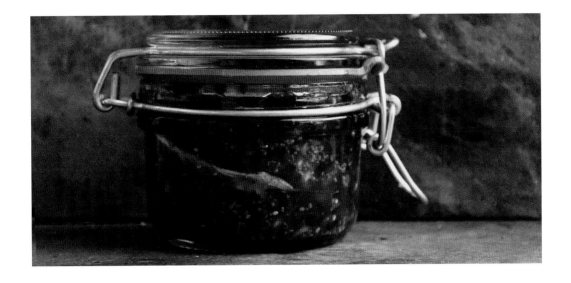

STONE-GROUND WILD BLACK MUSTARD

The hills around Los Angeles are loaded with this "invasive" mustard. It's highly edible, with a wasabi-like flavor profile, but very few people take advantage of this unwanted yet plentiful mustard. The plant is cultivated in North Africa (and probably other regions) for its black or dark brown seeds, which are used as a spice.

At the end of summer, it usually takes me 30 minutes to gather enough seeds to fill nearly 2 cups (180 g). You don't have to be a wildcrafter to make this mustard. You can find black mustard seeds in some specialty grocery stores (Middle Eastern or Indian) or online. But frankly, if you make this using wild mustard seeds, it will taste so much better than anything you can buy at the store. The flavor profile is between a Dijon mustard and wasabi paste—quite strong but delicious!

Ingredients for a 1-pint jar (480 ml) —around three-quarters full

½ cup (45 g) black mustard seeds
½ cup (120 ml) red wine vinegar, apple cider vinegar, or your own homemade vinegar
¼ cup (60 ml) white wine or beer
2 teaspoons (10 ml) honey or maple syrup
1½ teaspoons (7.5 g) salt

Procedure

Place the seeds in a stone grinder (molcajete) and add enough vinegar and wine to cover the seeds. Grind for 2 to 3 minutes, then let it rest for 5 minutes.

Add more vinegar and wine and repeat the process. You may need to do this 3 or 4 times. Once you have achieved the consistency you like, stir in the honey and the salt.

Transfer the mustard into a jar and place it in the fridge. The fresh mustard will be quite bitter. You'll need to age it for at least a week before using it. It will keep in the fridge for several months.

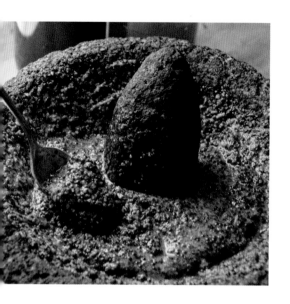

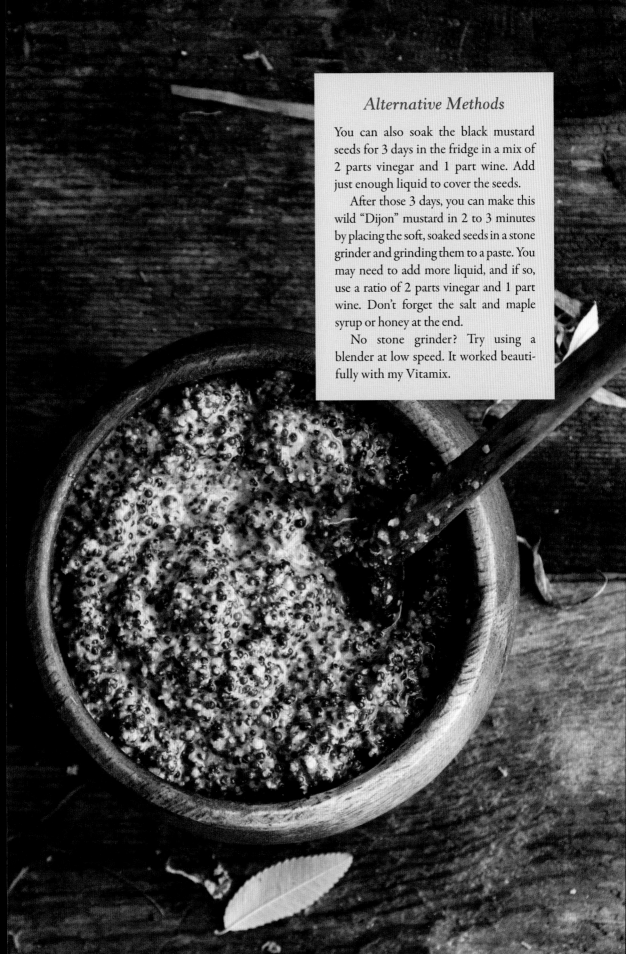

Alternative Methods

You can also soak the black mustard seeds for 3 days in the fridge in a mix of 2 parts vinegar and 1 part wine. Add just enough liquid to cover the seeds.

After those 3 days, you can make this wild "Dijon" mustard in 2 to 3 minutes by placing the soft, soaked seeds in a stone grinder and grinding them to a paste. You may need to add more liquid, and if so, use a ratio of 2 parts vinegar and 1 part wine. Don't forget the salt and maple syrup or honey at the end.

No stone grinder? Try using a blender at low speed. It worked beautifully with my Vitamix.

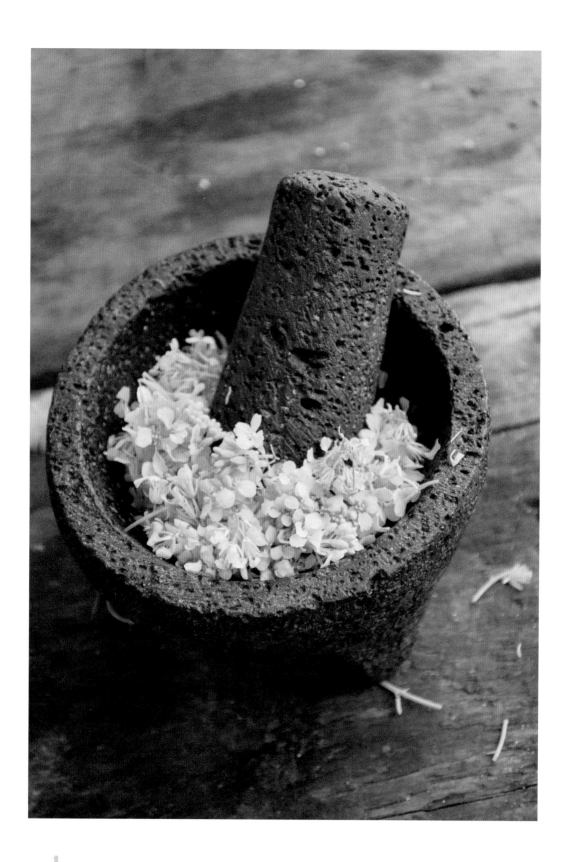

MUSTARD FLOWERS "WASABI"

Each year when the flowers are blooming, I make a potent "wasabi" sauce with local black mustard flowers. It's delicious with fish or fermented mushrooms, but it's also fantastic on toasts and sandwiches.

To make this black mustard "wasabi," you just need to collect very fresh black mustard flowers. Don't place the flowers in a plastic bag while foraging them—in my experience, they tend to ferment very quickly, probably due to the large amount of wild yeast on them. Collect them in a small cloth or canvas bag and hurry home. I often slightly wet my collecting bag, which helps keep the flowers cool and fresh.

This is really a gourmet condiment. The famed chef Niki Nakayama from n/naka restaurant (featured in the television series *Chef's Table*) has used a similar sauce with black mustard flowers and leaves. As this recipe demonstrates, many unwanted and invasive weeds can actually be prepared into gourmet foods.

Don't eat too much of this condiment on an empty stomach, as it can create a stomach upset. But this is probably the case with regular wasabi, too. The recipe doesn't work with other mustards—they don't have the wasabi quality that black mustard does.

Ingredients

1 ounce (28 g) fresh black mustard flowers

2 tablespoons (30 ml) unpasteurized apple cider vinegar (white wine vinegar, champagne vinegar, or Mugwort Beer Vinegar work very well, too)

2 teaspoons (10 ml) red wine or beer

¼ teaspoon (1.3 g) salt

Procedure

Grind all the ingredients together. I use my molcajete. It takes 3 to 4 minutes to grind all the ingredients to a pulp. You can use a blender, too. The sauce will keep for at least a week or so in the fridge. Canning it doesn't work—the heat will destroy the spiciness.

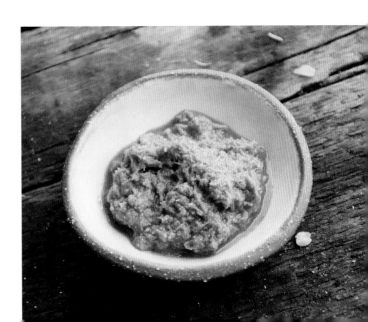

FOREST SALSA VERDE

Can you "taste" the forest in a salsa? With this recipe you can, and it's delicious. That's because this green salsa is made with herbs that can be collected from the forest floor.

The key is to use herbs that are quite flavorful. I'm lucky to have easy access to chickweed and wild chervil, which, as you'll have noticed by now, I use often. But you can use other savory wild herbs such as watercress, arugula, hairy cress (*Cardamine hirsuta*), perennial pepperweed (*Lepidium latifolium*), and so on. You can also substitute oxalis with young sorrel or unripe feral fruits such as apples in the northeastern United States, or with manzanita in California.

Think of this recipe as a concept and see what you can do with your terroir.

Ingredients for a
½-pint jar (240 ml)

1.5 ounces (43 g) mixed wild greens (about 40 percent chervil, 30 percent chickweed, 20 percent miner's lettuce, and 10 percent oxalis), see Note

1.5 ounces (43 g) jalapeño pepper

1.5 ounces (43 g) green bell pepper

0.5 ounce (14 g) red onion or shallot

2 tablespoons (30 ml) apple cider vinegar (beer or white wine vinegar, wild or not, works well, too)

1 tablespoon (15 ml) water or white wine (I've also used various wild fruit juices instead)

1 teaspoon (5 ml) maple syrup

¼ teaspoon (1.3 g) salt

> **Note:** *If you don't have wild chervil, you can substitute it with parsley or cilantro.*

Procedure

Clean the wild greens in cold water, then shake off the excess moisture. I often use my grandma's technique, which I call the "spinning towel":

> Lay a clean kitchen towel out flat.
> Place the wild greens in the center.
> Pick up the 4 corners in one hand to make a pouch.
> Go outside and swing in a wide circle for a few seconds.
> Return to the kitchen, open the towel, and remove the now dry wild greens.

Mince the wild greens and chop the peppers and onion. Mix all the ingredients together in a bowl.

I prepare the salsa 30 minutes before serving. During that time it becomes juicier, and the wild green flavors really start shining.

I like my salsas quite chunky, but if you want something that's smoother, you can just process all your ingredients in a blender for a minute or so and season to taste.

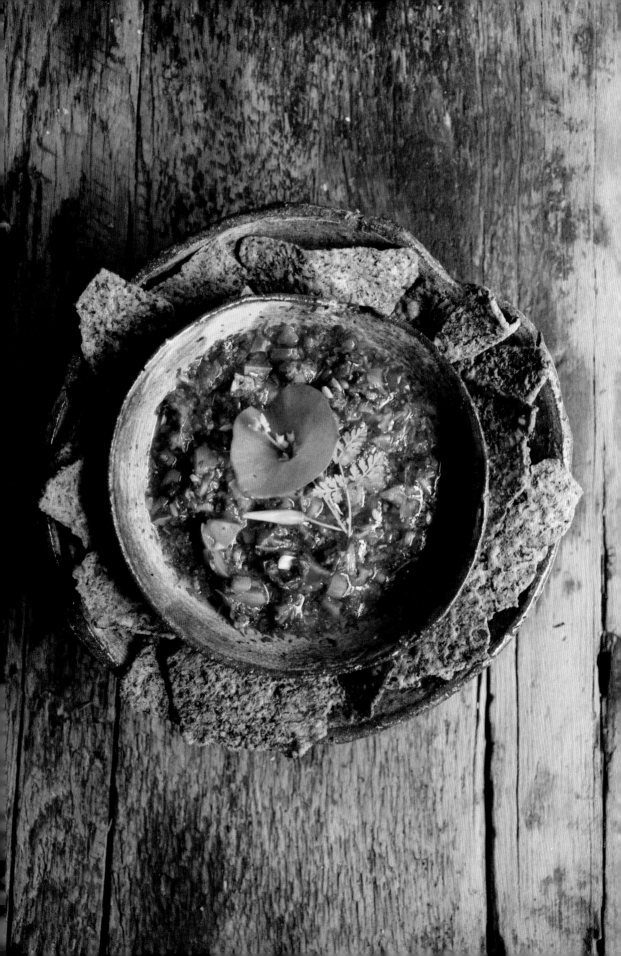

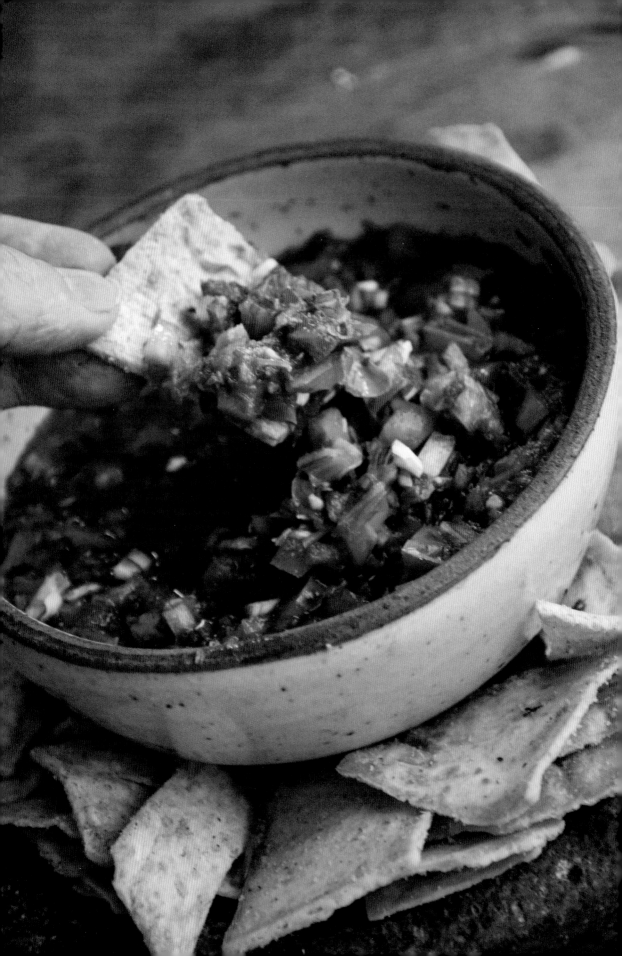

WILD FOOD SALSA

Add ingredients like tomatoes or red bell peppers to a Forest Salsa Verde and you end up with a more generic salsa. A true forest salsa recipe requires very savory ingredients to pull it off, but with a more generic salsa you can use milder ingredients like purslane, wild mustard(s), perennial pepperweed, or wild radish pods.

Of course, if you make your own vinegar, you can really make this wild food salsa shine. I've made it using some of my raw Apple Scraps Vinegar with a touch of Elderberry Wine Vinegar.

This recipe should give you around 1½ cups (360 ml) of salsa, which is perfect for 2 people. I like my salsa quite chunky, so I chop and mince by hand, but you can use a food processor or blender to make a smoother salsa.

Ingredients for 1½ cups (360 ml)

1.8 ounces (50 g) mixed wild greens (purslane, chickweed, chopped wild radish pods, sow thistle, perennial pepperweed, and chervil in this case)

½ green or red bell pepper (around 3.5 ounces or 100 g)

1 small tomato, diced (3.5 ounces or 100 g)

1.8 ounces (50 g) red onion

1.8 ounces (50 g) green jalapeño

⅓ cup (80 ml) unpasteurized apple cider vinegar

1 tablespoon (15 ml) maple syrup

½ teaspoon (2.5 g) salt

Procedure

Clean the foraged ingredients in cold water, then shake off the excess moisture. I often use my grandma's technique, which I call the "spinning towel," see page 148.

Mince the wild greens and chop the green pepper, tomato, onion, and jalapeño. In a bowl, mix all the ingredients together.

Let the salsa rest for an hour or so. It will last in the fridge for 2 to 3 days, but it's much better in terms of texture if you eat it within 24 hours.

ITALIAN SALSA VERDE: CHICKWEED AND WILD CHERVIL

In Italy, this type of sauce is mostly used with skirt steak or fish. It's also fantastic with pan-roasted potatoes or mushrooms.

Traditionally, lemon juice is used as an acid, but this is a good example of how a savory homemade vinegar can play this role and make a taste difference. In this case, I used my Smoked Mushroom Seaweed–Infused Vinegar.

It's a recipe to try with your local wild edibles, even if you don't have access to wild chervil or chickweed. You can use an herb such as watercress, or you can mix miner's lettuce with parsley and a bit of sweet white clover.

Ingredients

4 tablespoons (60 ml) olive oil

3 tablespoons (12 g) minced chickweed

3 tablespoons (45 ml) unpasteurized apple cider vinegar (or lemon juice or Smoked Mushroom Seaweed–Infused Vinegar)

2 tablespoons (8 g) wild chervil or parsley

1 tablespoon (4 g) capers, minced

1 tablespoon (4 g) chopped or minced jalapeño

2 garlic cloves, minced

½ teaspoon (2.5 g) salt

¼ teaspoon (1.5 g) ground pepper

½ teaspoon (1 g) chili flakes

4 to 5 green olives, minced (optional)

2 salted anchovy filets, minced (optional)

1 teaspoon (3 g) dried herbes de Provence or Italian herbs (optional)

Procedure

Simplicity itself—mix all the ingredients together and voila! I like to let the sauce rest for a few hours or even overnight in the fridge so all the flavors blend together nicely.

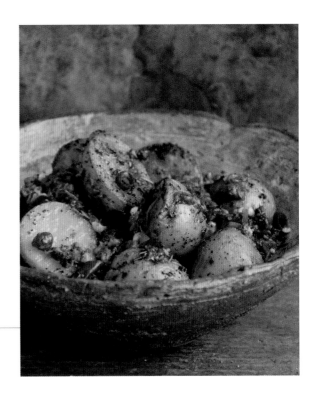

I often mix this Italian Salsa Verde with sauteed potatoes and serve it to my students after a class. It's always an instant hit.

Collecting Wild Seeds

Gathering wild seeds and grains was an important part of my routine when I was living in the Los Angeles area. For a wildcrafter, it might have seemed that there was nothing to forage, mostly because after summer the whole region would turn into a dried-up, desert like landscape.

But underneath that appearance, there was a true bounty of edible nutritious seeds and grains that could be collected for making mush (soft paste), adding to bread and crackers, sprouting, and creating condiments. Based on my research, there are probably around 200 edible seeds and grains in Southern California alone. Many of them are non-native and sometimes invasive.

I use several techniques to collect and process seeds. When dealing with a new plant, at least one of them usually works well.

Gentle Grinding

This grinding technique is used for seed pods that don't release their seeds easily. The idea is to place the plants or seed pods into a mortar or other hand grinder (I use my molcajete) and grind slowly to break down the chaff or pods. It's an exercise in gentleness, as you don't want to break the seeds or grains themselves. When finished, use a strainer to separate the grains from the pods or chaff. This method works well with curly dock, evening primrose (*Oenothera elata*), and cheatgrass (*Bromus tectorum*).

Feet Stomping

The feet-stomping technique is very efficient with plants from the mustard family, such as black or Mediterranean mustard. In late summer, break off the tops of the dried-up mustard plants when they are loaded with seed pods and stuff them into a plastic or paper bag. Once home, do a happy dance on the bag for a couple of minutes, which will break down the pods and release the seeds inside the bag. Rip a corner off and let the chaff and seeds fall out into a strainer placed over a bowl. The chaff will stay in the strainer, and you'll collect the seeds in the bowl. Super easy.

Passive Seed Collection

Nothing much to do with this method, but timing is important. Pick the plants when they're going to seed, rest them across a bowl or large plate. As they dehydrate, the seeds will automatically fall. It's a good method for chickweed, lamb's-quarter (*Chenopodium album*), some grasses, and the like.

Seed Drop from Living Plants

Let nature do the work. Collect the plants when they're just going to seed. Place them into a vase with water. Place a paper underneath the vase to collect the seeds as they fall off the plant. This is the perfect technique for plants like miner's lettuce that drop their seeds within a few days.

Shaking

I mostly use this shaking technique for sages and my local wild chia. Bring a large bowl or paper bag with you into the field. Shake the seed pods and let the seeds drop in the bag.

Hand extraction

Without the proper equipment, sometimes you're stuck having to remove grains by hand. This is especially true for wild oats or barley. There are no modern tools to remove cheatgrass grains, so if I want them perfect, I'll put some calming ambient music on and get to work. It takes a lot of time, but I find it very meditative.

Roasting and Burning

I haven't yet tried this method, but I plan to do it with wild oats and other grains that I otherwise need to extract by hand. In North Africa, a traditional method of grain extraction is to roast and burn green wheat (durum wheat, *Triticum durum*), then rub it to extract the grains. The result is a cereal food called *freekeh* or *farik* in Arabic.

This method is dependent on timing—the grains should be close to maturity but not fully ripe. The green wheat is cut, piled, and sun-dried, but not to the point that the unripe grains inside have lost their moisture. The pile is then set on fire so only the chaff and straw burn. The roasted grains are removed by rubbing or threshing, then sun-dried.

A similar technique, called *Grünkern*, was used in Germany.

I think it's worth exploring this technique with some wild grains and seeds—it could make the job easier and impart some smoky flavors.

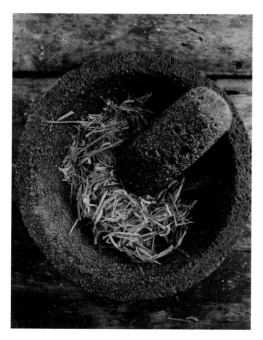

Grinding. Gently roll the pestle to break down the seed pods. Use a strainer to separate the seeds later on.

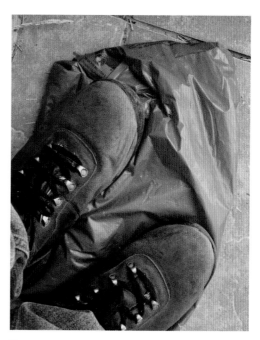

Feet stomping. Do a little dance on a bag stuffed with seed pods. Rip a corner to strain the chaff and collect the seeds.

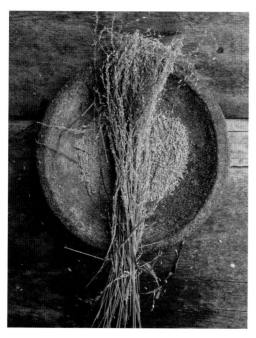

Passive seed collection. Dehydrate and let the seeds or grains drop into the container.

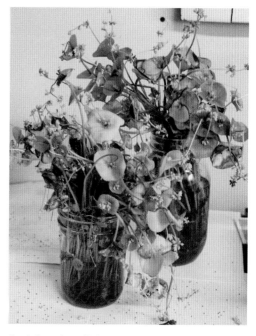

Seed drop from living plants. Collect plants going to seed and place them in a vase with water. Place a paper underneath and simply wait.

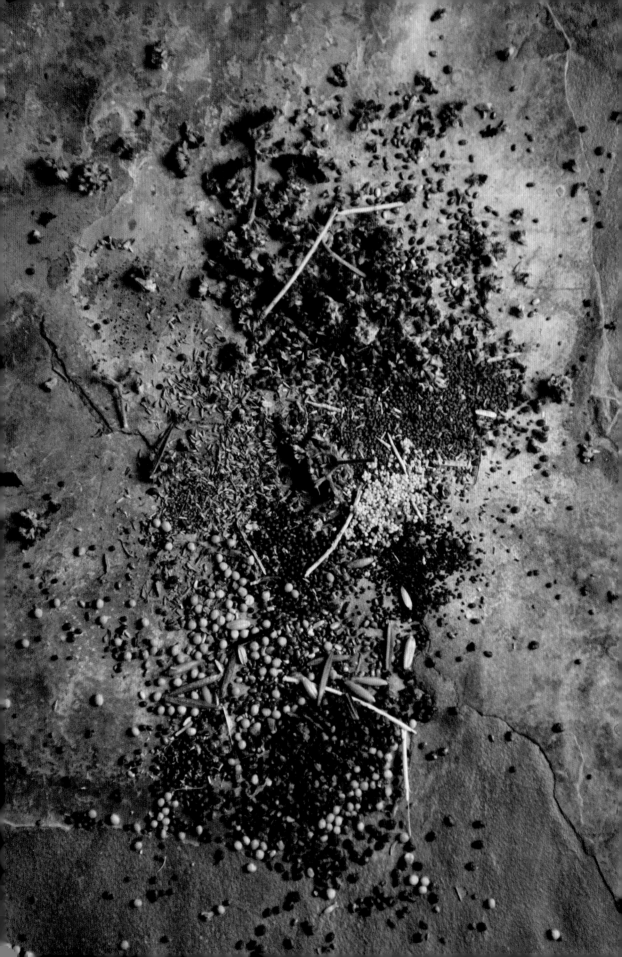

Storing Seeds and Grains

Many of the wild seeds and grains you forage will still have a decent amount of moisture inside. Before you store them in a closed container, you'll need to make sure they are dehydrated enough.

I had to learn that the hard way. The first time I foraged black mustard seeds, I immediately stored them in closed jars and within a couple of weeks I had a moldy mess inside. My whole harvest for that year was lost.

These days, my usual method is to store seeds or grains in paper bags for at least a couple of months before transferring them to a closed jar or similar container. Another method is to place your seeds and grains in a jar with a paper towel secured on top with a rubber band. After a couple of months, remove the paper towel and replace with the tightly sealed lid.

I use my wild seeds and grains within a couple of years.

Some of the foraged seeds I've used for pickling include:

Black mustard
Mediterranean mustard
Broadleaf plantain
   (*Plantago major*)
Black sage
Wild chia
London rocket (*Sisymbrium irio*)
Narrowleaf plantain
   (*P. lanceolata*)
Wild fennel
Lamb's-quarter
Field mustard (*Brassica rapa*)
Common stinging nettles

Curly dock
Chickweed
Wild chervil
Wild oat
Sunflower (*Helianthus* spp.)
White sage
Evening primrose
California buckwheat
   (*Eriogonum fasciculatum*)
Miner's lettuce
Sedge (Cyperaceae family)
Wild celery
Cheatgrass

PICKLED WILD SEEDS

This is a mustard-like condiment I make yearly using foraged seeds. The culinary uses are similar to regular mustard; I use it in salads, sandwiches, with cheese, and so on. The recipe will change based on what's available in any given year and where you happen to be, but you can also do something similar with store-bought seeds. The only common denominator is that I use black mustard seeds as my base—they're quite spicy and will make this condiment taste like a cross between Dijon mustard and wasabi.

If you can't find black mustard seeds in your environment, black and yellow mustard seeds can be purchased in specialty grocery stores (Middle Eastern and Indian) or online. Apple cider vinegar works well with this recipe, but my Mountains Vinegar really brings it to a new level. I used to make a large quantity every year for a local Michelin-starred restaurant. I make a point of using a lot of invasive plants I find locally. Basically, I am removing unwanted weeds and turning them into gourmet food instead of using herbicides to eradicate them, which poison the ground. I like positive solutions!

I don't have a precise recipe, so think of this as a concept. The last batch I made, which consisted of seeds collected in Southern California, Wyoming, and Colorado, was as follows here.

Ingredients for a 1-pint jar (480 ml)

2.5 ounces (70 g) black mustard seeds

1.25 ounces (35 g) yellow mustard seeds

1 tablespoon (9 g) Mediterranean mustard seeds

1 teaspoon (3 g) Asian mustard seeds

2 teaspoons (6 g) wild chia seeds

1 teaspoon (3 g) broadleaf plantain seeds

1 ounce (28 g) various edible wild seeds from the following plants: common stinging nettle, lamb's-quarter, curly dock, sedge, black sage, wild fennel, chickweed, wild chervil, and sunflower

1 cup (240 ml) unpasteurized apple cider vinegar (I use my Mountains Vinegar), more if needed

1 teaspoon (3 g) herb blend such as Italian herbs or herbes de Provence (optional)

1½ tablespoons (23 ml) maple syrup

½ teaspoon (2.5 g) salt

Procedure

Place all the seeds in a pint jar. You should end up with a half-full jar of seeds. Add the vinegar, herb blend, salt, and maple syrup. The ratio is about 50 percent seeds to 50 percent vinegar and syrup.

Close the jar and shake it at least once daily for the first 3 to 4 days. The seeds will swell and you will end up with a thick, caviar-like condiment. The chia and broadleaf plantain seeds will make it quite mucilaginous. During the first two days, as the seeds absorb the vinegar, you can add a small amount of vinegar to achieve the consistency you like.

Store in the fridge. It should last for at least 6 months.

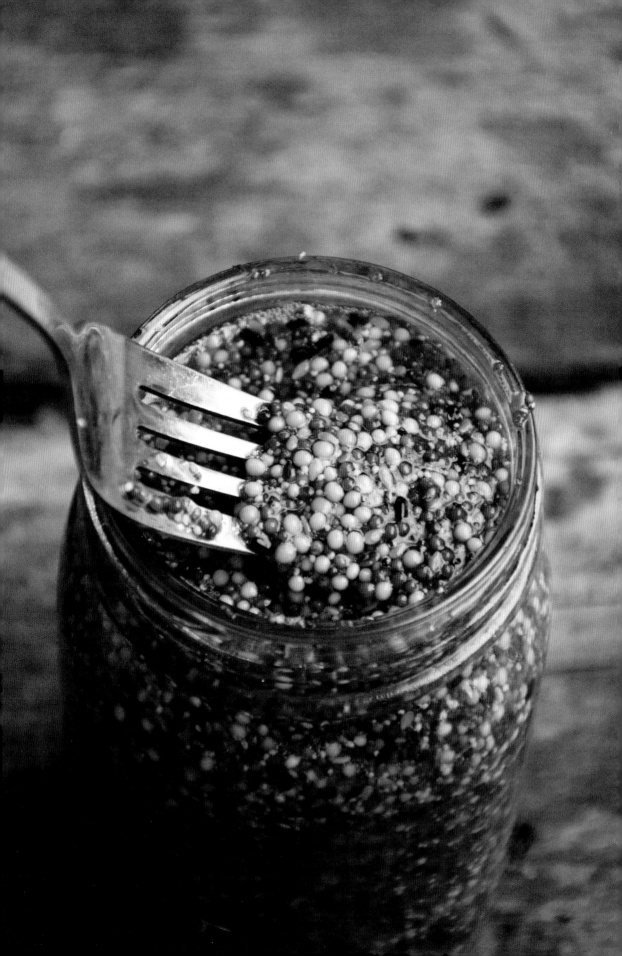

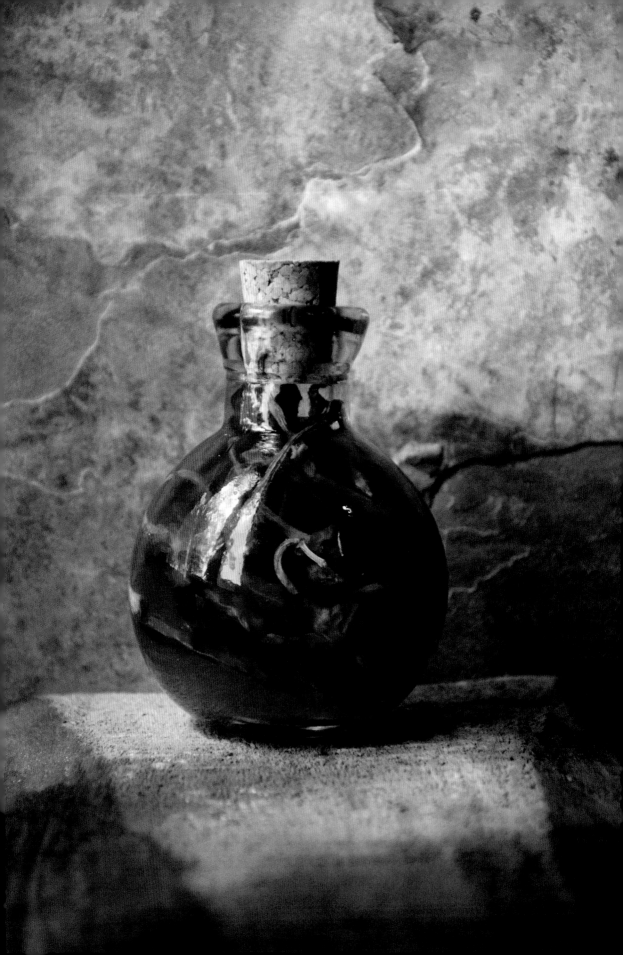

CHAPTER 5

Hot Sauces and
Fermented Spicy Vinegars

There is a deep association between hot sauces and vinegars. I simply could not live with myself if I wrote a book about vinegar and didn't include a chapter about hot sauces and similar spicy concoctions. It just wouldn't be right.

I'm a big fan of hot sauces. Every couple of weeks I must purchase a new one and try it. While the flavors of a good hot sauce are mostly based on the choice of peppers and added spices or herbs, if you make homemade vinegars from scratch, you will find that vinegar can add a spectacular new dimension.

The vast majority of commercial hot sauce recipes use distilled white vinegar as a base. It makes sense in that context, as white vinegar is quite cheap and has a somewhat neutral flavor. Some artisanal sauces use apple cider vinegar or wine vinegar, which adds some sweet and fruity accents.

If you are a homemade vinegar aficionado and decide to experiment with hot sauces, you'll quickly realize that vinegar itself can be one of the main flavor components. For example, a couple of weeks ago I made a somewhat mild hot sauce using mostly dried chile pasilla (chile negro), a small amount of chile morita (smoked jalapeño peppers), brown sugar, homemade sea salt, and a touch of garlic powder. That recipe would make a decent sauce with regular vinegar, but you can go so much further!

Chile pasilla is rich in fruity flavors with chocolaty and woody tones, while chile morita packs a decent amount of heat and has a definite smoky accent. To complement the fruity flavors, I decided to use some of my Elderberry Wine Vinegar as the base. The result was quite amazing, a wonderful harmony of sour, sweet, spicy, salty, fruity, and smoky. It would have been impossible to achieve this with a regular vinegar.

You can make hot sauces using different methods and ingredients such as:

Hot sauces using fresh peppers, herbs, and spices

Hot sauces using dried peppers, herbs, and spices

Hot sauces using chili powders and spices

Hot sauces using both fresh and dried ingredients

Lacto-fermented hot sauces with fresh and dried ingredients

Spicy, vinegar-based pastes

Most store-bought hot sauces are usually red or green, but because we're dealing with wildcrafted or homemade vinegars, we'll explore creating dark burgundy and even whitish hot sauces.

As always in my books, there are no rules. If you are an experienced wildcrafter, hot sauces are another medium for exploring the true flavors of your local terroir. Aside from using vinegars made from foraged fruits and berries, you can also add local herbs, spices, barks, mushrooms, pine needles, and so on.

Let's explore the possibilities!

How Spicy Is It?

The Scoville scale is a measure of how spicy a chili pepper tastes. "Heat" is measured in Scoville Heat Units. Originally, spiciness was determined by taste alone, which was somewhat subjective, but these days it is determined by a measure of capsaicinoid levels. Capsaicinoids are the chemical compounds responsible for the heat we feel when eating peppers. Capsaicin is the main component of this compound.

Table 5.1 features the most common chili peppers that can be purchased commercially or sometimes found in the wild (such as chiltepin peppers and pequin peppers). The competition to create the hottest peppers is quite fierce, and every couple of years another one seems to break the record. Most of them are not readily available at your local store but can be purchased online. Personally, although I love some good heat, I think habanero is spicy enough.

Bottled Pain: Chili Pepper–Infused Vinegar

This recipe is very simple. Although it's essentially just dried peppers placed in vinegar, it's another example of how a good homemade vinegar can make a huge difference in terms of flavors.

Table 5.1. Spiciness of Common Chili Peppers

Scoville Heat Units	Pepper
3,180,000	Pepper X
1,569,300–2,200,000	Carolina reaper pepper
1,463,700	Trinidad scorpion
1,382,118	Naga viper pepper
1,041,427	Naga bhut jolokia pepper
100,000–350,000	Habanero
100,000–325,000	Scotch bonnet
100,000–225,000	Birds eye pepper
100,000–125,000	Carolina cayenne pepper
50,000–100,000	Thai pepper
50,000–100,000	Chiltepin pepper
40,000–58,000	Pequin pepper
30,000–50,000	Cayenne pepper
30,000–50,000	Tabasco pepper
15,000–30,000	de Arbol pepper
6,000–23,000	Serrano pepper
5,000–10,000	Chipotle pepper (smoked ripe jalapeño)
5,000–10,000	Chile morita (lightly smoked ripe jalapeño)
2,500–5,000	Jalapeño
1,000–2,000	Chile ancho
1,000–2,000	Poblano pepper
1,000–2,000	Chile negro (also called chile pasilla)
1,000–1,500	Korean chile pepper
500–2,500	Chile California
500–2,500	Anaheim pepper
500–1,000	New Mexico pepper
0	Sweet bell pepper

Yes, you could make this using white vinegar or other store-bought vinegars, but you just can't compare those results with the flavors you'll achieve using your own vinegar.

The process is very straightforward—place a bunch of dried chili peppers in a bottle and fill it up with vinegar. Infuse it for 3 to 4 weeks, then strain and bottle. You can also place the original (unstrained) container in the fridge and enjoy it all year long. It gets spicier with time.

Simple enough, but let's go a bit further. You can use this uncomplicated process to create a delicious masterpiece in a few different ways:

Use your own homemade vinegar or infused vinegar. I have made this infusion using my homemade Smoked Mushrooms and Seaweed–Infused Vinegar, Mountains Vinegar, and Blackberry Wine Vinegar.

Think of it as a double flavor extraction. The first extraction occurred in the original infused vinegar, and the next one is the chili pepper infusion.

Of course, you can decide to mix everything together from the beginning (seaweed, mushrooms, and chili peppers) as you'll see in another recipe shortly.

Choose your chili peppers. Chili peppers can be spicy, sweet, toasted, or smoked. Did you know that through selective breeding and hybridization, there are tens of thousands of chili pepper cultivars available today? When I was living in Los Angeles, the number of different varieties was mind-boggling. My favorites were chile morita (smoked ripe red jalapeño peppers), ancho chile, and black chili pods. Some chilies will benefit from a little bit of pan-toasting (2 to 3 minutes) to bring out the savory and aromatic oil. You can also create tasty blends that don't need to be very spicy.

Add spices or wild aromatic herbs. My last batch had a tiny touch of curry, coriander, and peppercorn.

Add sugar and salt. Most people omit this part, but a good balance of sweetness and saltiness can add another dimension to your spicy creation. I often use my regular seasoning recipe, which is:

¼ cup (60 ml) homemade vinegar
2 teaspoons (10 ml) maple syrup or honey
½ teaspoon (2.5 g) salt

There is no specific recipe for this chili infusion, just guidelines. It's up to you to create your own masterpiece!

Using Dried Chili Powder

Probably one of the easiest ways to make a hot sauce is to use chili powders, which can be purchased. If you have your own garden, you can grow your own peppers, dehydrate them, then make your own savory and spicy

powders using a coffee grinder (or stone mortar). You can even mix different types of chili peppers.

Some hot sauces you find in the supermarket are made with only powdered ingredients, vinegar, and salt. Many years ago, I tried to make hot
sauces that way. I ended up with mixed results. My main problem, which I
didn't realize at the time, was the fact that I never diluted the vinegar; thus,
the acidity was a bit overwhelming. Most hot sauces made with chili powder use a ratio of 1 part vinegar (at 5 percent acidity) to 1 part water. You
can't go wrong with that ratio.

I'm a little different because a lot of my hot sauces are also meant to feature the special flavors of the homemade wildcrafted vinegars I make. My
ratio of vinegar to water is slightly higher. A typical recipe looks like this:

⅔ cup (160 ml) vinegar
⅓ cup (80 ml) water
3 to 4 tablespoons (18 to 24 g) chili powder
½ teaspoon (2.5 g) salt

And of course, you have the optional additions, wildcrafted or not,
which can really make your sauce unique: onion powder, curry, cumin, wild
aromatic herbs (sages, sagebrush), California bay, sumac, dried basil, dried
oregano, wild tarragon, and more.

You're also not stuck with using water to dilute the vinegar. I've made
hot sauces using fruit juices from blackberries, cactus pears, and elderberries (you'll need to boil the juice for elderberries) instead of water.

I hope this makes you realize that you have *a lot* of creative possibilities.

HOT SAUCE WITH DRIED CHILI POWDERS

If you've never made a hot sauce with powdered ingredients before, let's get started with a very simple recipe and a typical procedure.

Ingredients for one 5-ounce bottle (148 ml)

1 tablespoon (9 g) chipotle powder (see Note)
1 tablespoon (9 g) paprika powder
1 teaspoon (3 g) garlic powder
½ teaspoon (1.5 g) ginger powder
⅛ teaspoon (0.25 g) curry powder (optional)
½ teaspoon (2.5 g) salt
¼ cup (60 ml) unpasteurized store-bought apple cider vinegar or ⅓ cup (80 ml) homemade vinegar with at least 5 percent acidity
¼ cup (60 ml) water
1 tablespoon (15 ml) maple syrup, sugar, or honey

Procedure

In a pint (480 ml) jar, mix the various powders and salt with a spoon.

Add the vinegar, water, and maple syrup. Seal the jar and shake well for a couple of minutes. Transfer the contents into the 5-ounce (148 ml) bottle and store it in the fridge. Wait 2 to 3 days before using the sauce—this will allow the flavors to blend. The sauce will keep for several months in the fridge.

Note: If you want your sauce to be spicier, you can use 2 tablespoons (18 g) of chipotle powder instead of 1 tablespoon (9 g).

Xanthan Gum

You often need to shake hot sauces made with powdered ingredients before using them, as some of the powders will tend to settle at the bottom. If this bothers you, you can remedy this problem with the addition of xanthan gum.

Xanthan gum is a food additive that is used as a thickener and stabilizer. If you look at the labels and ingredients on most commercial hot sauces, you'll find it listed. The gum is a manufactured product made from fermented sugar with the bacteria *Xanthomonas campestris*. Although you won't find the gum in nature, it's not "unnatural" per se.

There are natural thickeners that can be used instead, such as arrowroot powder or corn starch, but you'll need to heat the sauce first to use them. The advantage of xanthan gum is that you can use it with a cold liquid. Add the gum powder once your hot sauce is ready. Make sure you stir it vigorously while adding the powder slowly, or better yet, add it while blending the sauce so it doesn't form clumps.

You don't need a lot—use ¼ teaspoon (0.5 g) for every 1 quart (1 L) to start. The higher the amount of gum powder you use, the thicker the sauce will become.

Pasteurization

If you want to gift some of your hot sauces to friends, I suggest pasteurizing them. It makes sense from a food safety perspective, as you don't know how they will store your gift. A couple of months ago, I visited a friend and found a bottle of hot sauce on the shelf with the cap loosely placed on top. The ambient temperature was around 85°F (30°C), and who knows how many weeks or months that bottle had been stored there. In terms of food safety, heat and oxygen are not your friends.

There are several methods to pasteurize the sauce and the bottles—all of them can be found with a little bit of online searching. You can also find pasteurization guidelines among the USDA recommendations related to canning. One of the most common methods is as follow:

1. Sterilize your bottles by filling a canner or large pot with water.
2. Bring the water to a rolling boil. Add the bottles and make sure that they are fully submerged.
3. Leave the bottles for 10 minutes in boiling water, then remove.
4. Meanwhile, heat the sauce to 180°F (82°C) for 10 minutes (make sure to stir), then immediately transfer the sauce into your sterilized bottles.
5. Screw the caps on tight. Turn the bottles upside down for at least 10 minutes; this will sanitize the lids.

MOUNTAINS HOT SAUCE

This is a hot sauce I made for one of my wild food tasting workshops. It incorporates ingredients from the local mountains around Los Angeles and, of course, uses the Mountains Vinegar as the foundation of the sauce, which is infused with over 15 plants, berries, and even mushrooms from the same location.

This hot sauce is so hyperlocal that you could not make it outside of Southern California, but no matter. Use this recipe and apply it to where you live—you can create something unique to your region with a little bit of research and experimentation.

I make this sauce in 2 parts. The first part is very similar to the basic recipe for making Hot Sauce with Dried Chili Powders. In the second part, I soak the dried berries, seeds, and herbs in hot water for 30 minutes to help extract their flavors.

Ingredients for two 5-ounce bottles (296 ml)

½ cup (120 ml) Mountains Vinegar
1½ teaspoons (4 g) ginger powder
½ teaspoon (1.5 g) curry powder
1 teaspoon (3 g) garlic powder
1 tablespoon (9 g) chile morita powder
1½ tablespoons (13.5 g) smoked paprika powder
½ cup (120 ml) water
¼ cup (60 ml) blackberry juice
2 large (0.4 ounces, or 12 g) chile pasilla (also called chile negro)
2 tablespoons (15 g) cracked and stone-ground manzanita berries
1 tablespoon (6 g) dried elderberries
1 tablespoon (15 ml) pinyon pine cone syrup
1 fermented lime (0.2 ounces, or 5 g) (also called loomi)
1 yarrow flower
1 teaspoon (3 g) black mustard seeds
½ teaspoon (0.7 g) dried sweet white clover
½ teaspoon (2.5 g) sea salt
½ teaspoon (1.5 g) sumac powder
¼ teaspoon (0.5 g) xanthan gum

Procedure

1. Pour the vinegar into a pint (480 ml) jar, then add the following powders: ginger, curry, garlic, chile morita, and smoked paprika powder. Stir with a clean spoon.
2. In a saucepan, combine all the other ingredients aside from the xanthan gum.
3. Bring the contents to a boil and immediately turn off the heat. Let the contents cool for around 30 minutes.
4. Strain the contents of the pot into the pint jar containing the vinegar and powders. Shake well.
5. Pour the hot sauce into a blender and blend at medium speed. Slowly and carefully add the xanthan gum.
6. Transfer to the 2 clean 5-ounce (148 ml) bottles. You should have enough sauce to fill 2 bottles.
7. Place in the fridge and wait 3 to 4 days before using. This will allow the flavors to blend together well. Your sauce will keep for at least 6 months in the fridge.

Note: I've introduced smoky flavors to this sauce by adding roasted oak bark to the pint jar and aging it in the fridge for 3 weeks before transferring the contents to bottles. Of course, you also have the option of adding a small amount of "liquid smoke," which can be found at your local supermarket.

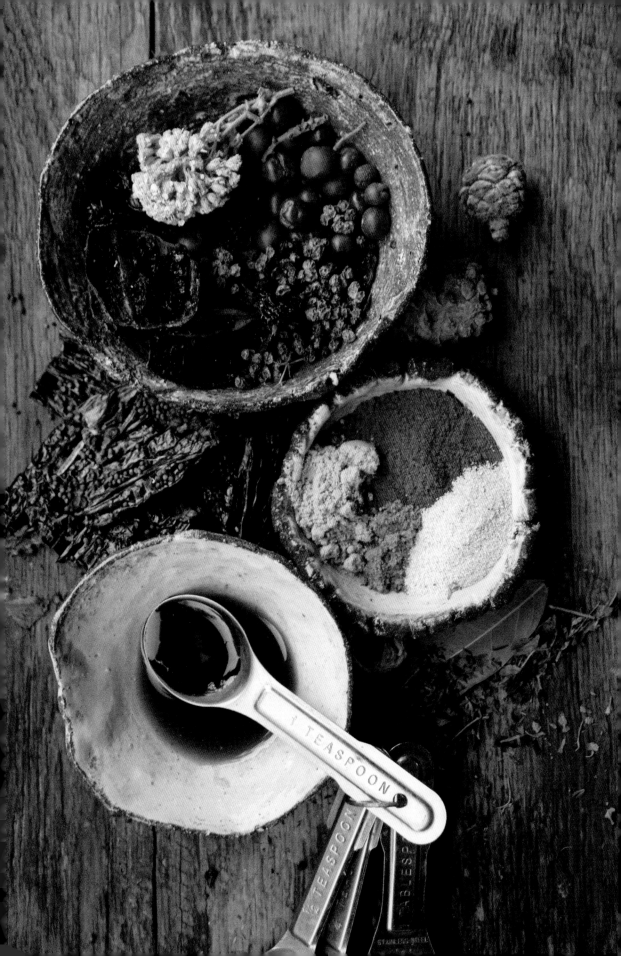

HOT SAUCE FROM
DRIED CHILI PEPPERS

You can make very creative blends and delicious hot sauces using dried chili peppers. I like to use sweet and tasty peppers like chile pasilla or ancho as a base, then add more spicy ones like chile morita (smoked jalapeño peppers).

To extract the oils and flavors, we'll first toast the dried chili peppers in a pan for a couple of minutes. With experience, you can do it by smell. Some people remove the seeds, as they can give a slight bitter edge, but I use everything.

Ingredients for a
½-pint jar (240 ml)

3 to 4 dried chile pasilla (0.6 ounces, or 16 g) (you can also use chile ancho)

3 dried chile California (0.6 ounces, or 16 g)

2 chile morita (0.2 ounces, or 6 g)

1 cup (240 ml) unpasteurized apple cider vinegar or red wine vinegar (I love using my Elderberry Wine Vinegar for this recipe)

½ cup (120 ml) water

2 tablespoons (30 ml) maple syrup, honey, or sugar

2 teaspoons (6 g) garlic powder

1 teaspoon (3 g) ginger powder

1 teaspoon (5 g) salt, more if needed

Procedure

1. Pan roast the chili peppers to your liking, then place all the ingredients in an uncovered saucepan. Bring the contents to a slow simmer for 15 minutes.

2. Let it cool for 5 minutes or so, then transfer to a blender.

3. Process until you get the consistency you want. Sometimes I like my sauce to be chunky, but if you plan to bottle it instead of storing it in a jar, you might prefer a very smooth sauce. Taste and add more salt or sugar if desired.

4. Pour the sauce into the jar, close the top, and store in the fridge. It will keep for months.

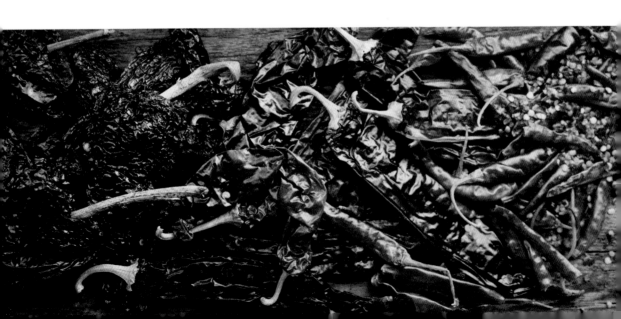

HOT SAUCE WITH COOKED CHILI PEPPERS

This recipe will allow you to explore and start experimenting with your own local wild food. I make it quite often for my wild food tasting events. Instead of fresh parsley I use local savory wild herbs such as chickweed, miner's lettuce, wild chervil, curly dock leaves, small amounts of oxalis, and so on.

This sauce is great with river or lake fish such as trout, tacos (plant-based or not), wild food salad, and countless other dishes.

A good homemade apple cider vinegar or white wine vinegar will work beautifully.

Ingredients for an 8-ounce bottle (240 ml)

8 ounces (227 g) jalapeño peppers (around 6 large jalapeños)

1.8 ounces (50 g) chopped onion (around ⅓ of a medium onion)

1 garlic clove, chopped

1 to 2 teaspoons (5 to 10 ml) olive oil

⅓ cup (80 ml) apple cider vinegar

¼ cup (60 ml) water

1 teaspoon (3 g) dried Italian herbs or herbes de Provence (optional)

1 tablespoon (15 ml) maple syrup

1 teaspoon (5 g) salt

½ teaspoon (1.5 g) ginger powder

¼ teaspoon (0.5 g) ground black pepper

0.7 ounces (20 g) parsley, cilantro, or mixed wild herbs, chopped

Xanthan gum (optional), see Note

Procedure

Clean the jalapeños and remove the stems. I usually cut them lengthwise and remove the seeds.

In a stainless steel or similar nonreactive pan, sauté the chopped onion and garlic with the olive oil until slightly browned.

Add the sliced jalapeños and the rest of the ingredients, except for the parsley or other fresh herbs, and simmer for around 5 minutes.

Transfer to a blender and add the parsley.

Process to the desired consistency, chunky or thin, then transfer the contents into the bottle.

Store in the fridge where it will last for months.

Note: *Without xanthan gum, you'll need to shake the container before serving. If you want to add xanthan gum, add it slowly to the blender at low speed. Use a ratio of ¼ teaspoon (0.6 g) gum for 1 quart sauce (1 L) to start. The higher the amount of gum powder, the thicker the sauce will become.*

DRIED CHILI PEPPERS AND
WILDER FLAVORS

There are lots of ingredients in this sauce, but it's a good example of how you can use foraged berries and plants to create sauces that become a reflection of your terroir.

It's quite similar to the procedure in Hot Sauce from Dried Chili Peppers, but I'll break the rules a little by adding ingredients that can be used for flavoring but will need to be removed prior to blending and processing the sauce.

Ingredients for a
½-pint jar (240 ml)

0.6 ounces (16 g) dried chile pasilla
  (or chile ancho)
0.6 ounces (16 g) dried chile California
0.2 ounces (5 g) dried chile morita (see Note)
1¼ cups (300 ml) red wine vinegar
½ cup (120 ml) blackberry juice
2½ tablespoons (37 ml) maple syrup,
  more if needed
2 teaspoons (4 g) dried elderberries
2 teaspoons (6 g) ground dried
  manzanita berries
1½ teaspoons (7.5 g) salt, more if needed
2 teaspoons (6 g) garlic powder
1 teaspoon (3 g) peppercorn
1 teaspoon (2.5 g) wild sumac
  (or commercial sumac powder)
1 teaspoon (2 g) grated ginger
¼ California bay leaf or ½ regular bay leaf

Procedure

1. Pan roast the peppers to your liking, then place all the ingredients in an uncovered saucepan.
2. Bring the contents to a simmer for 15 to 20 minutes, then let it cool until lukewarm (15 minutes or so).
3. Carefully remove the peppers and place them in a blender. Strain the rest of the concoction, then add the liquid into the blender, as well.
4. Process until you get the consistency you want. Sometimes I like my sauce to be a bit chunky, but if you plan to bottle it instead of storing it in a jar, you might prefer a very smooth sauce.
5. Taste and add more salt or maple syrup if you want.
6. Pour the sauce into a jar or bottle, close the top, and store in the fridge. It will keep for months.

Note: This sauce is not spectacularly hot. Double the amount of chile morita if you like more heat and wildcrafted pain.

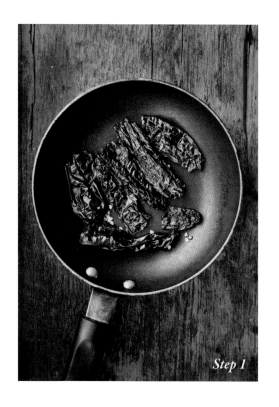

Step 1

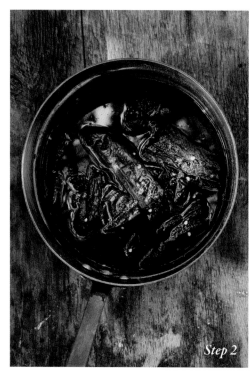

Step 2

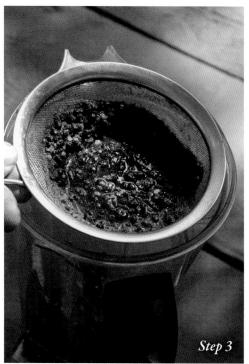

Step 3

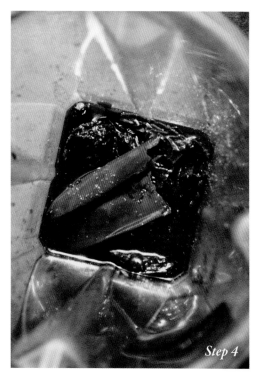

Step 4

Hot Sauces and Fermented Spicy Vinegars | 173

RAW HOT SAUCE

You can make a basic raw sauce using ingredients similar to those in the Hot Sauce with Cooked Chili Peppers, but skip the onion or use less, as some people who are sensitive to them may experience digestive problems when they aren't cooked.

A raw sauce is perfect in early spring. I make this type of sauce a day before a wild food class and use a mix of foraged herbs such as watercress, chickweed, miner's lettuce, and so on.

You can use a homemade red wine vinegar or any wild (red) berry wine vinegar (blackberry, elderberry, and the like) with red peppers, or a good apple cider vinegar with green peppers. A red vinegar with green peppers will make your sauce look muddy.

Feel free to mix peppers for optimum flavors and heat.

Ingredients for a 1-pint jar (480 ml)

8 ounces (227 g) fresh chili peppers
½ cup (120 ml) apple cider vinegar
   or red wine vinegar
¼ cup (60 ml) water or apple juice
2 garlic cloves
1 ounce (28 g) chopped wild greens,
   parsley, or cilantro
1 tablespoon (15 ml) maple syrup
1 teaspoon (5 g) salt
1 teaspoon (2 g) grated fresh ginger

Procedure

Clean the peppers and remove the stems. Cut them lengthwise and remove the seeds if desired.

Place all the ingredients in a blender and process to the desired consistency, chunky or thin. You also have the option of straining the sauce.

Transfer the contents into a jar, bottle, or similar container. Close the top and store in the fridge where it will keep for at least a week.

Note: For flavor and color, if you make a red pepper sauce, you can also add a couple teaspoons of smoked paprika or mild chili powder.

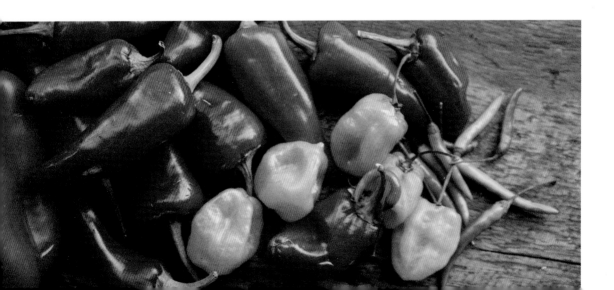

FERMENTING A PEPPER MASH: TABASCO-STYLE HOT SAUCE

One of my favorite hot sauces is Tabasco. It's a simple vinegar-based sauce with a nice kick, and I'd always wanted to create something similar but spicier by using one of my favorite chili peppers: habanero.

And so, a couple of years ago, I invested some time and did a bunch of research on fermented hot sauces and the basic method behind making Tabasco.

To keep it super simple, Tabasco is made from a tabasco pepper mash that is lacto-fermented with salt and aged for 3 years in toasted barrels. After 3 years, the fermented mash is removed from the barrels and mixed with distilled vinegar in a stainless-steel tank using a ratio of 30 percent mash and 70 percent vinegar. The contents are stirred daily and aged for another month or so, strained, and bottled. That's it!

To ferment a pepper mash, you just need salt. The *Lactobacillus* bacteria responsible for the fermentation process are already present on the ingredients you are using. Fermentation is an anaerobic process, and most books will tell you that you have to keep the ingredients that you are using under the brine. That's true for fermented ingredients like carrots or whole peppers, but the problem with liquid ferments such as hot sauces or salsas is that you can't really keep the ingredients under a brine. There is a higher risk of spoilage because the top of the ferment will be in contact with oxygen, which can promote the growth of "bad" bacteria or mold.

But it's not an issue if you work with your ferment. The solution is to stir or shake the contents daily. I do it at least once a day until the initial fermentation is done, and the contents are acidic enough to inhibit the growth of

unwanted bacteria or mold. You'll know the initial fermentation is done when you don't have any substantial fermentation gases being released inside the jar, and therefore very little or no pressure on the closed lid (see "Using Lids as Pressure Gauges," page 178). I've never had any mold or spoiling issues using this method.

Another thing to know is that a pepper mash requires more salt than your average lacto-ferment because peppers are more prone to molding. The consensus is that one should use between 5 and 10 percent salt by weight.

I usually use about 5 percent, which is around 4 teaspoons (20 g) of salt per pound (455 g) of ingredients used for the mash.

You'd better wear gloves! I once made a large quantity of hot sauce without using gloves. My peppers were super hot and it ended up being quite a painful experience that lasted hours, thanks to the capsaicin.

Procedure for Fermented Pepper Mash

1. Gather all the pepper mash ingredients and chop them crudely.
2. Place pepper mash into a bowl. Weigh the contents. Based on the weight, calculate the amount of salt you want to use, which is usually between 5 and 10 percent of the weight of the ingredients.

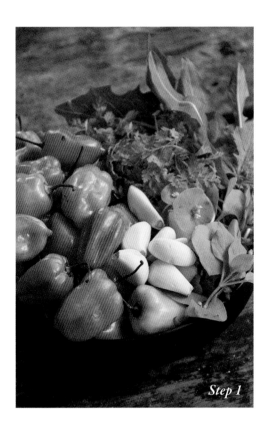

Step 1

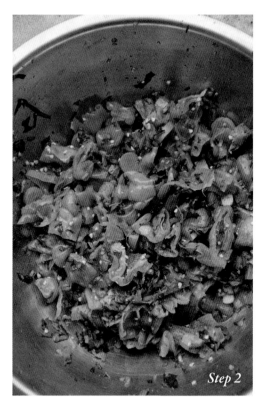

Step 2

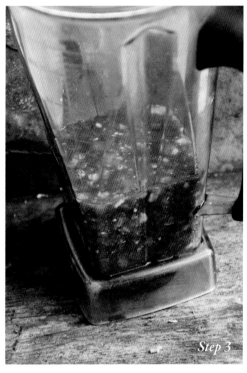

Step 3

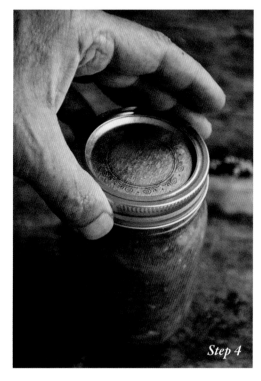

Step 4

3. Transfer the contents into a food processor, then add the salt. Blend to the consistency you like.
4. When done, pour the contents into a clean jar, no more than three-quarters full. Close the lid, but not too tight so the fermentation gases can escape. (See Note.)
5. A couple of times a day, screw the lid on tight and shake the contents for a few seconds, then unscrew the lid just a tad. As an alternative, if the sauce is too thick, you can also open the jar, stir briefly with a clean fork or spoon, then screw the lid back on (not too tight).
6. Ferment your pepper mash for at least 2 to 3 weeks or more. After that period, close the lid and place the jar in the fridge if desired. I've also fermented hot sauce pepper mash for months at room temperature, stirring the contents maybe once a week.

For pepper mash ferments, don't fill the jar more than three-quarters full, as sometimes bubbles created during the fermentation process will push the ingredients upward. Not a problem if you monitor your ferment during the day, but I've had a couple of occasions when I woke to a mess due to a very active fermentation during the night.

As I wrote earlier, Tabasco pepper mash is aged for 3 years in toasted barrels. You don't have to wait that long. The whole process usually takes 3 weeks and, if I recall correctly, the longest time I've aged a pepper mash in a glass jar was 2 months in a cool, dark place (a closet).

Note: *If you work at home like I do, as an alternative you can close the lid tight and burp it (open it briefly to let the pressure off) at least once daily or more as necessary. With experience you can feel how much pressure is generated by the ferment in the jar by pressing the lid. Burping 1 to 3 times a day is necessary for the first 10 days, and then usually once daily after that. Over time the fermentation gases will slow down considerably, and the contents will be acidic enough that mold won't be an issue.*

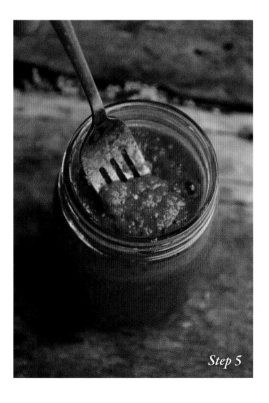
Step 5

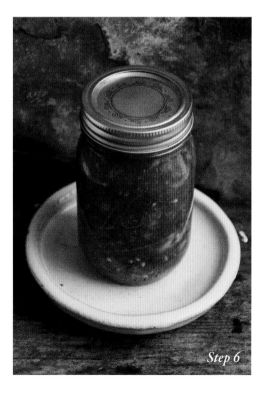
Step 6

Using Lids as Pressure Gauges

Fermenting in mason jars with closed lids is a bit controversial in fermentation circles, but it really isn't too risky if you have experience and carefully monitor your ferments. I would not advise you to do it if you're new to fermenting—it's probably better if you unscrew the lid a bit so fermentation gases can escape. But otherwise, closed lids are an interesting tool for determining if a ferment is active or not.

When a lid is screwed tight, the fermentation gases can't escape and create internal pressure, which will push the lid upward. With experience, by pressing on the lid with your index finger, you can gauge how active a ferment is. If the pressure is excessive, you can "burp" the jar by unscrewing the lid, and from there you can decide to leave the lid unscrewed a bit so fermentation gases can escape, or to close it again if you want to monitor the pressure further.

Please note that it takes discipline and constant monitoring (sometimes several times a day) to use this method. If you're a forgetful-type person, it's not for you. Neglecting a very active ferment for a day or two can either create a mess or can be downright dangerous. Your lid will either bend and pop out of the jar with force, lots of liquid or fermenting ingredients will burst out (which is usually what happens), or the jar will explode. Jar explosion is rare but can occur. You really need to supervise and "burp" them every day to release the pressure.

Using the lid as a gauge is also useful for determining if an initial fermentation, usually around 10 days, is done. I often close the lid when I think it's finished and check the pressure at the end of the day or the next day. If there is barely any pressure or none, I know it's time to place my jar in the fridge for aging.

Personally, I find this method quite helpful and I use it a lot. But as I said earlier, it's much better if you're an experienced fermenter and you know you have the discipline necessary to monitor your ferments daily. When done responsibly, there is also something very personal about this approach—it really helps you establish a close relationship with your ferments.

Checking the pH

If you start doing lacto-fermentation experiments such as adding wild edibles, making low-salt ferments, or fermenting unusual ingredients such as mushrooms (remember to cook them), it's a *very* good idea to invest a bit of money and purchase a pH meter. They are useful if you deal with pastes or hot sauces.

A good quality pH meter used to be quite expensive, but these days you can buy one for less than $20 online. A pH meter will give you a reading on the pH scale, which measures how acidic or basic a substance is. The pH scale ranges from 0 to 14. The lower the number, the more acidic the ingredients are. For example, vinegar has a pH level of around 3. A sauerkraut or kimchi is usually around 3.3.

The pH is important to know because of one specific bacterium, *Clostridium botulinum*. The spores of this bacterium are found in soil and on the surface of some ingredients such as roots, fruits, and vegetables. *C. botulinum* thrives in certain anaerobic environments. It can lie dormant for years, but under the right conditions, such as the absence of oxygen in a jar, the spores may grow out into active bacteria again, producing neurotoxins in the process. The resulting poisoning from ingesting contaminated ingredients is called botulism, which can be fatal. Even when treated, it is fatal for 5 to 10 percent of people in developed countries. Untreated, you have a 50 percent chance of death. Not something to sneer at.

But, on the positive side, *C. botulinum* cannot grow below a pH of 4.6, which is one of the reasons why fermentation works so well. Ferments such as sauerkraut, kimchi, or a basic pepper mash will quickly reach an acidity well below 4.6, thus making botulism a nonissue.

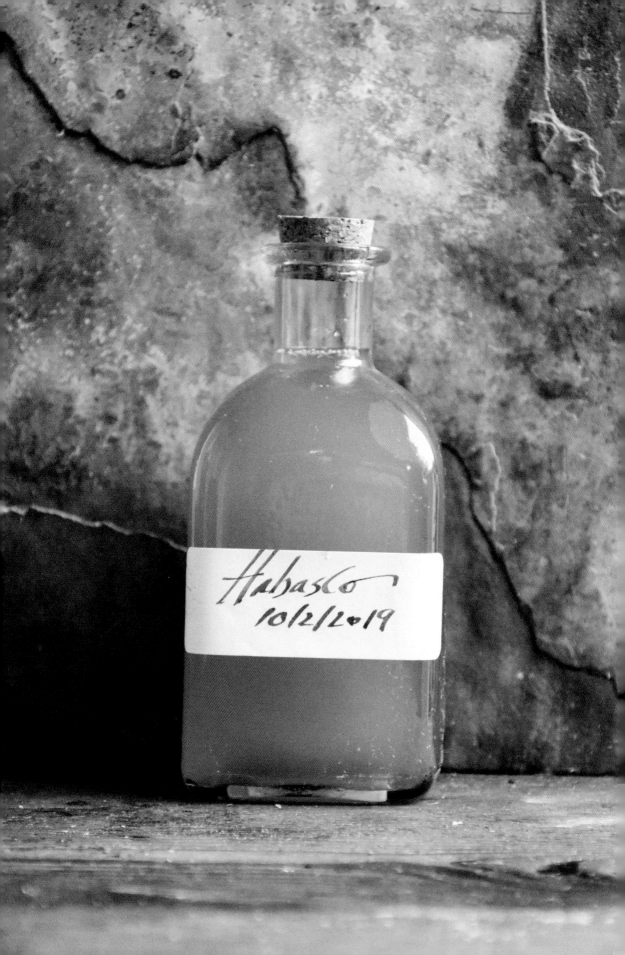

HABASCO: FERMENTED HABANERO HOT SAUCE (TABASCO-STYLE)

You don't need to be a fermentation expert to make this kind of sauce. This is really a basic lacto-fermentation process. You can try this recipe with other peppers, such as cayenne or serrano.

Before you panic at the idea of using mostly habaneros, you should know that the fermentation process will bring down the heat. It will still be spicier than a regular Tabasco sauce, but it's deliciously survivable.

The culture starter is optional, but I often add it to ensure success.

Ingredients for a 1-quart jar (1 L)

13 ounces (368 g) fresh habaneros
½ cup (120 ml) water, more if needed
15 garlic cloves, peeled
2½ ounces (70 g) mixed wild edibles
5 tablespoons (37.5 g) mild chili powder (I use Korean chili powder)
3 pieces (1 inch, or 2.5 cm, each) of roasted oak bark (optional)
2 tablespoons (30 ml) culture starter (sauerkraut or kimchi juice or whey) (optional)
Salt (5 to 10 percent of the total weight after blending the above ingredients)
Raw or pasteurized apple cider vinegar (I use my Mountains Vinegar); see ratio used in the procedure

Procedure

Place everything except the salt, bark, and vinegar into a blender and make a rough paste. Transfer the contents into a bowl and add the salt. Stir the contents to make sure the salt is dissolved properly then transfer to a jar. You can add more water if the paste is too "solid," but not much.

At this point I also like to add a bit of roasted oak bark after blending for a smoky touch. The oak will impart flavors, as well.

Close the top or screw the lid, but not too tight. A couple of times each day, close the lid tightly and shake the jar for a minute or so (so you don't get mold on top). You can also stir the contents with a fork or spoon. Burp as necessary. After around 2 to 3 weeks, once the initial fermentation is complete and there are no more fermentation gases, stir the contents once or twice a week. Age at room temperature for anywhere between 1 week to 2 months.

Transfer to a larger jar and add the vinegar. I keep the ratio at 30 percent fermented sauce and 70 percent vinegar, around 2¾ cups in this case.

Shake the contents once daily for 3 weeks, then strain. Voila! Your own habasco! Taste, cry, and add more salt if you want. The one I'm enjoying right now was bottled 6 months ago.

Spicy Vinegar from Fermented Roots

I've always been fascinated by roots. They're usually not high on the list of wild food priorities, but although hidden from sight, they can be magnificent in terms of taste.

Southern California was far from the land of known edible roots, although after many years of exploring the land and with some experimentation, I had success with many roots from the Brassicaceae family and a few others.

In the Los Angeles area, I was able to find around 8 different types of edible wild mustards, all of them non-native and some considered invasive. Unlike young wild radish roots, mustard roots are too stringy and tough to eat as is, but if you scrape one with a knife and smell it, you'll realize there is a whole universe of pungent earthiness and deliciousness in there. This is especially true for black mustard and Mediterranean mustard roots, which have some definite horseradish and wasabi qualities.

The main issue was to find a way to extract those earthy flavors. After doing all kinds of experiments, I finally found a good one. The secret to extracting flavors from such tough, stringy roots is lacto-fermentation.

The procedure is quite simple. I thoroughly clean the foraged roots (I use a toothbrush) in cold water. Next, I cut them into smaller pieces with a pruning shear or crush them in a molcajete, then I ferment them in brine (salted water) with added spices. I use a tratio of 1½ to 2 teaspoons (7.5 to 10 g) of salt per cup (240 ml) of water. You can also add the spices as you crush the roots.

Usually, in fermentation, you keep the ingredients under the brine, but for this preparation I fill only half the jar with my spicy brine. I think the flavors are more concentrated if I use less brine. To avoid any spoilage issues, all you need to do is shake your concoction several times daily and burp as necessary. When the initial fermentation is done—around 2 weeks—you can strain the flavored brine and use it in soups, sauces, and other condiments.

As I was making some Tabasco-like hot sauces, I realized they would be a perfect use for my fermented mustard roots. I was not wrong! I added more heat (hot chili peppers) to the original fermented root recipe and used less brine. Once the fermentation was complete, I filled the jar with homemade apple cider vinegar and aged the contents for a month or so.

By the way, while there aren't many edible roots in Southern California, there quite a few throughout North America and Europe. These include wild carrots, Queen Anne's lace, burdock (*Arctium* spp.), prairie turnip (*Pediomelum esculentum*), purple poppy mallow (*Callirhoe involucrata*),

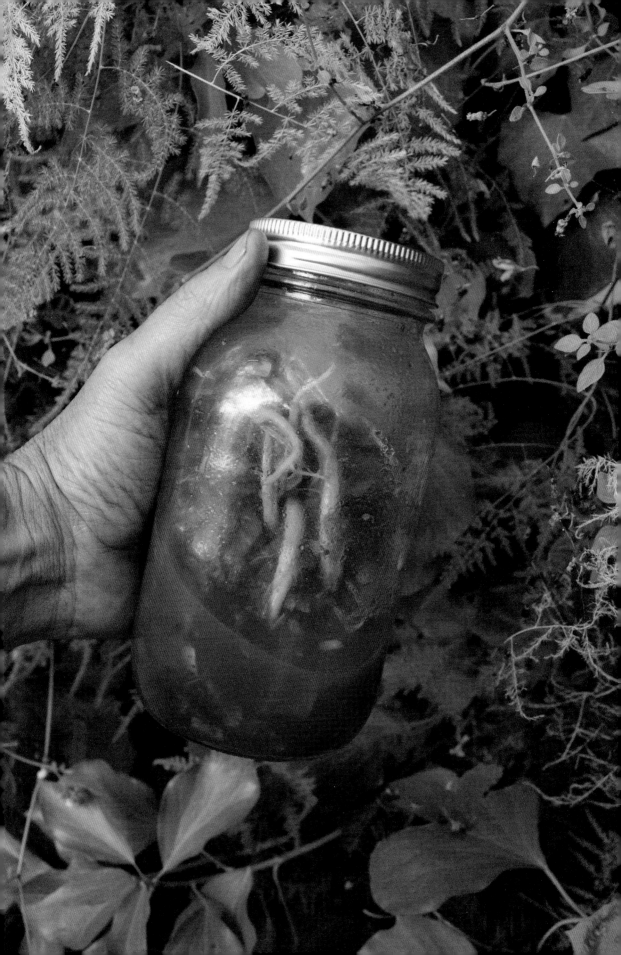

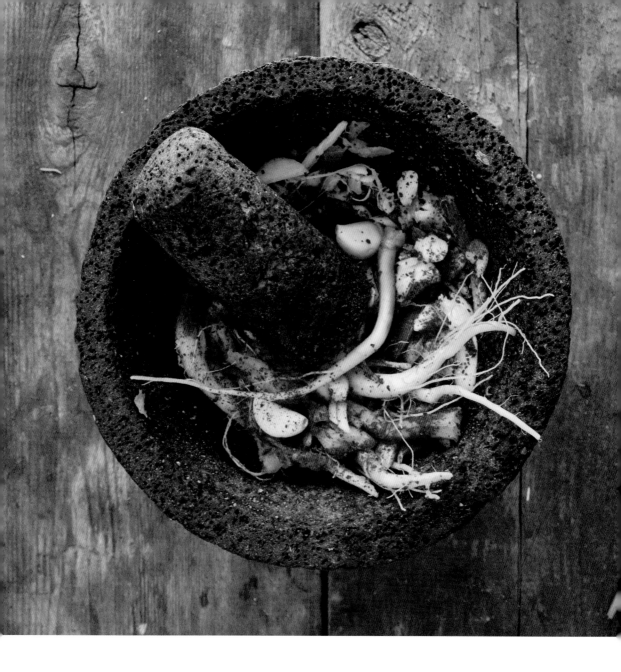

creeping bellflower (*Campanula rapunculoides*), and many others. I recently spent time in Colorado, where I made a similar spicy ferment using burdock roots. The end result was quite awesome.

If you think about it, roots are a new way to look at the wild edibles you may already know. Examine the roots, scrape them with a knife, and smell or chew on them. Do some thorough research on edibility before making any elaborate ferments. That said, the mustard family is usually safe. For some practical advice to get you started, see "Infusing Whole Environments" on page 116.

FERMENTED MUSTARD ROOTS HOT SAUCE

This method can be used with roots that have interesting flavors but are too tough and considered "inedible" due to their texture, including mustard roots and wild radish roots.

The procedure has two stages. First you ferment the roots in brine, and then you add the vinegar and age the contents. In my book *Wildcrafted Fermentation*, this kind of ferment was used to make soup stocks. In this case we're making a spicy vinegar, so we'll add more "heat" and use a smaller amount of brine.

Ingredients to ferment in a 1-quart jar (1 L)

6 ounces (170 g) wild radish roots (or more)
12 to 15 garlic cloves
2 to 3 tablespoons (18 to 27 g) spicy chili flakes or powder (I use chile morita)
1 cup (240 ml) water (not tap water) divided
1½ to 2 teaspoons (8 to 11 g) salt

Procedure

Clean your foraged roots in cold tap water. Don't use hot water, as this may kill the lactobacteria present on the roots.

Using a molcajete, crush the roots and garlic cloves by pounding them, then put them in a separate bowl. If you don't have a stone grinder, a hammer or stone on a hard surface should work.

In the bowl containing the crushed roots and garlic, add the chili flakes and ¼ cup (60 ml) of the water (not tap water, which contains chlorine). Mix everything well.

Note that instead of using a separate bowl, you also have the option of placing all the ingredients so far in the molcajete and making a splendid mess by pounding everything together.

Transfer all the ingredients into the jar.

Make a brine with the rest of the water (¾ cup, or 180 ml) and the salt, then pour it into the jar and close the lid. The brine will reach up to around one-third of the jar's volume. That's okay—I do that on purpose to concentrate the flavors in the brine.

A couple of times daily, burp the contents (unscrew the lid a bit so the fermentation gases can escape) and shake for a few seconds. By doing so, you distribute the acidity that arises from the fermentation process, reducing the possibility of mold or rotting. But you need to have the discipline to shake at least daily. Another option is to close the lid, but not so tightly that fermentation gases can't escape if the pressure is excessive. You'll still need to shake the jar a couple of times daily.

The initial fermentation usually takes 10 to 15 days depending on temperature. You'll know it's done when there are no more fermentation gases. If you want, you can place that ferment in the fridge and age it for a few weeks or a couple of months.

Making the Spicy Vinegar

To make the spicy fermented roots into hot sauce, all you need to do is to add enough vinegar to fill the jar containing the fermented roots and brine. A good homemade apple cider vinegar works well with this kind of sauce.

Shake the contents a couple of times daily for a month, then strain.

That's it! It's that simple and delicious.

If you are an experienced fermenter, you can explore an incredible number of creative possibilities by mixing lacto-fermentation and vinegar fermentation. I've barely scratched the surface.

CHAPTER 6

Wildcrafted Appetizers and Side Dishes

This chapter is a chapter of ideas. I call it that because there are truly no limits on the number of tasty side dishes and appetizers you can create using your homemade vinegars and wildcrafted (or not) ingredients. With the addition of vinegar, most edible plants, berries, mushrooms, roots, and even seeds can be preserved, or their flavors can be elevated. You have thousands of ingredients to play with.

When we have a wild food tasting event after one of my plant walks or foraging workshops, I would say that around 30 percent of the tasting dishes use vinegar in some way, usually in the form of quick pickles. And I'm also not shy about mixing lacto-fermented ingredients with vinegars.

From my perspective, creating small dishes for people to sample is the best way to introduce them to wild edibles. One could write several books about examples of wildcrafted side dishes and appetizers—probably one large book for every state in North America and every country in the world.

It's possible to delve extremely deep into local flavors that are impossible to obtain through the regular food system. For example, try going to the supermarket to purchase the ingredients to make fermented and marinated pheasant's back mushroom (*Cerioporus squamosus*) with seasoned Elderberry Wine Vinegars and wild garlic. It's just not possible.

There is a true artistry, both in terms of flavor and aesthetic, in creating the right combination of ingredients and blending of flavors. Vinegar allows you to satisfy all the savory tastes: sweet, sour, spicy, bitter, and salty.

In this chapter, I've tried to include basic recipes for all the major groups of ingredients that can be found in the wilderness and then used to create side dishes or appetizers. We're talking roots, mushrooms, seeds, grains, nuts, stems, flower buds, and so on. But think of these recipes as concepts and ideas. I'm sure that, using your own local resources and personal

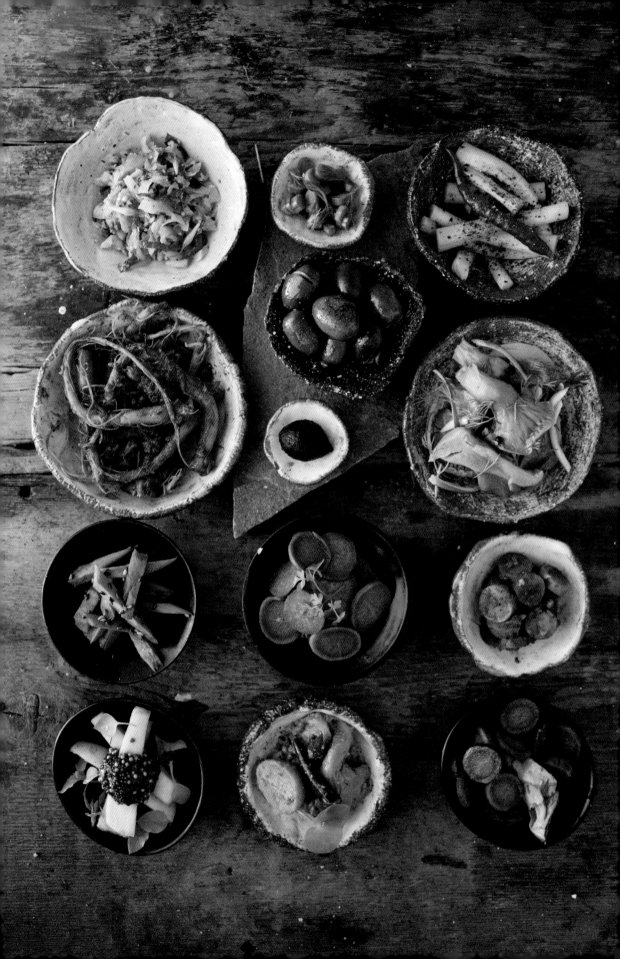

inspiration, you can create innovative, beautiful, and delicious side dishes and appetizers that are savory masterpieces.

Quick Pickling

Quick pickling is one of the easiest ways to preserve (wild) food for a relatively short time. Another name for quick pickles is refrigerator pickles.

Through the use of homemade vinegars, you can turn quick pickles into truly gourmet offerings, and if you are a wildcrafter, you can feature some of your local wild food and create interesting and tasty side dishes.

Think pickled wild radish pods or roots, mustard leaves, burdock roots, mallow or black mustard stems, wild onions, cooked mushrooms, and so on. You can also quick pickle regular ingredients, such as cucumbers, seasoned with tasty foraged herbs like wild fennel or dill weed.

The beauty of this preservation method is that you don't have to wait long before eating the pickle—usually a few hours or days. You also don't need any special equipment or an understanding of more complex preserving methods like canning.

Quick pickles are simply vegetables, roots, fruits, or mushrooms that are preserved in vinegar, water, salt, and sometimes sugar. To create quick pickles you'll need to follow a basic brine formula—about 50 percent vinegar and 50 percent water. This ratio is not set in stone, and you can adjust it based on your preferences. Most quick pickles will last for up to 2 months in the refrigerator, but long-term aging may alter the texture. For example, I would not keep quick pickled onions or shallots for more than 2 weeks.

Since I make a lot of unusual wildcrafted vinegars which are, by themselves, an excellent source of flavor, I often use more vinegar than indicated in the basic brine formula. For example, the brine for my last quick pickle (mushrooms) was composed of around 70 percent vinegar and 30 percent water.

Quick pickles can be highly creative and beautiful. There are several factors that can truly make a pickled side dish shine: the choice of vinegar, the amount of salt and sugar, the type of spices, how the ingredients are cut up, and how long it is aged.

Vinegar

Vinegar often takes backstage in online quick pickle recipes, which is rather strange because we're talking about preserving *in vinegar*. But it makes sense too, because most people purchase their vinegar from the store; thus, these recipes mostly call for white vinegar or apple cider vinegar.

Homemade vinegars can really add a new savory dimension. In my humble opinion, infused vinegars are the best! If I quick pickle cucumber slices with dill, but instead of using white vinegar or apple cider vinegar I use my Mountains Vinegar or my smoked Seaweed-Infused Vinegar, this simple side dish becomes spectacular.

Pairing the vinegar with the ingredient is important. For example, a pickled fish can be paired beautifully with a Seaweed-Infused Vinegar, whereas an Elderberry Wine Vinegar doesn't work as well, flavor-wise.

Salt and Sugar

It's not a must, but adding salt and sugar to balance the sourness of the vinegar can make a whole world of difference. It's also an easy way to boost the flavors of the other ingredients. Both salt and sugar are known as taste enhancers (umami).

Try the regular ratio I use, which is:

> 4 tablespoons (60 ml) homemade vinegar
> 2 teaspoons (10 ml) maple syrup or honey
> ½ teaspoon (2.5 g) salt

But remember, it's not a must. Some quick-pickled sweet fruits may not need any sugar or salt. You have to think like an artist and decide if or how you want to balance, subdue, or enhance the flavors.

Spices

Wild spices and savory herbs or leaves can be added to the pickling solution or sprinkled on the pickles just before serving. I add spices to most of my pickled creations. My wild spices include sages, California sagebrush, mugwort, wild fennel, white fir or spruce needles, dill weed, California bay leaves, and countless other foraged ingredients. Of course, I also use basic spices like coriander seeds, garlic, onion, thyme, basil, peppercorns, and so on. You can also use herb or spice blends such as Italian herbs, herbes de Provence, curry, and the like.

When available, I often add fresh minced herbs like chickweed, chervil, or fennel just before serving the side dish.

Knife Cut

Properly presenting your quick-pickled side dish is important. I always say that the aesthetics are at least 20 percent of the flavor. If something is beautiful, you're eager to try it. The proper knife cut is part of that aesthetic, and also makes the pickle easier to consume. For example, cucumbers are much better sliced than cut in large chunks.

The correct knife cut is also dictated by the texture of the ingredient used. For example, burdock roots are somewhat tough, and therefore much better when served in thin slices or cut into "fries." Herbs can be thinly minced, but fennel or dill fronds are better when crudely chopped.

It's something to keep in mind when you play with wild ingredients—how to plate them and what knife-cutting technique is the best to use.

Aging

From a food safety perspective, quick pickles can last a couple of months in the refrigerator. However, that doesn't mean this amount of time is best for all quick-pickled ingredients. My quick-pickled sliced cucumbers can be crunchy for a couple of days, but after 2 months their texture is terrible. Meanwhile, tough burdock roots benefit from a longer aging period.

To give you another example, I like my quick-pickled wild radish pods to be fresh, juicy, and crunchy; thus, my maximum aging period is around 2 to 3 days.

You'll need to experiment, and with experience you'll know what to do.

QUICK-PICKLED CUCUMBER CHIPS
AND WILD FENNEL

This is probably the easiest recipe in this book, and it's so good and refreshing. This humble dish is also a wonderful way to feature foraged greens that are packed with flavor, such as wild fennel or dill weed, which, as its name indicates, is considered a weed in areas like Colorado.

Ingredients for a 1-pint jar (480 ml)

8 ounces (227 g) cucumber,
    cut in ¼-inch (0.6 cm) slices
1 teaspoon (5 g) salt
½ cup (120 ml) raw apple cider vinegar,
    red wine vinegar, or Mugwort
    Beer Vinegar
½ cup (120 ml) water
1 tablespoon (15 ml) maple syrup,
    honey, or white sugar
2 teaspoons (1 g) minced fresh (or dried)
    wild fennel or dill fronds
¼ of a small red onion, chopped
½ of a garlic clove, minced (optional)

Procedure

Mix the cucumbers and salt together in a bowl. Let the contents rest for 10 minutes or so.

Meanwhile, combine the vinegar, water, and maple syrup in a separate dish. If you used sugar instead of maple syrup, stir the contents for a minute to dissolve the sugar.

Put the fresh minced fennel, onion, and garlic (if using) in a clean pint (480 ml) jar, then carefully place the cucumber slices inside the jar. You need to leave around ¾ inch (2 cm) headspace.

Pour the seasoned, diluted vinegar in the jar and make sure it covers the cucumber slices. Place in the fridge. It will keep for a couple of weeks, but it's much better (and crunchier) within 2 to 3 days. By the way, I often eat this side dish after marinating it for a couple of hours—it's quite fantastic when super fresh.

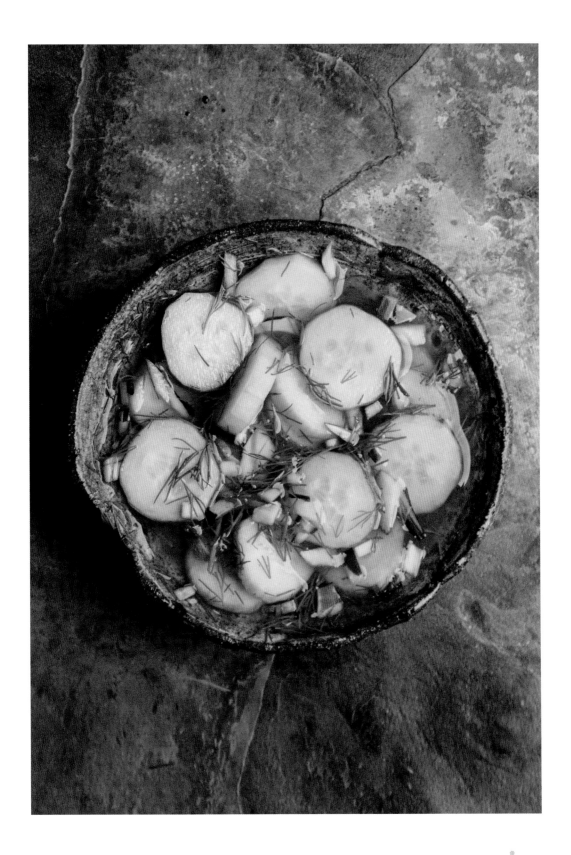

QUICK-PICKLED
BLACK MUSTARD LEAVES

This is a great little side dish. The recipe should work very well with a few other edible wild plant leaves, too, such as wild radish, perennial pepperweed, other types of mustard, and lamb's-quarter. I tried different traditional methods for pickling mustard greens and settled on the ones that called for boiling the leaves first. In terms of texture, it is necessary to boil our local black mustard or perennial pepperweed leaves, which would end up too chewy otherwise.

Ingredients for a
½-pint jar (240 ml)

8 ounces (227 g) black mustard greens

3 tablespoons (45 ml) raw apple cider
    vinegar (I use my Mountains Vinegar)

1 tablespoon (15 ml) water or white wine

2 teaspoons (10 ml) maple syrup,
    white sugar, or honey

½ teaspoon (1 g) chili flakes

½ teaspoon (1 g) grated fresh ginger (optional)

½ teaspoon (2.5 g) sea salt

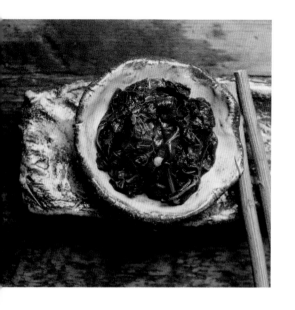

Procedure

Clean the greens, remove the stems, and, if you're using black mustard, remove the tough main vein that runs down the middle of the leaves. In a medium pot, bring around ⅓ gallon (1.25 L) of water to a boil and place the mustard leaves inside. Stir gently and remove the leaves after 1 minute, moving them to a bowl of cold water.

In a bowl, prepare the vinegar brine by mixing all the other ingredients. Stir well to dissolve the maple syrup and salt.

With clean hands, remove the boiled leaves from the cold water and squeeze them hard to remove the water. Chop the tight clump of leaves into ½- to 1-inch (1.3- to 2.5-cm) pieces.

Pack the leaves into the ½-pint (240 ml) jar, combine with the brine, and then place it in the fridge. You can eat the contents whenever you want, but it's much better after a couple of days. It will keep well for a month.

Some traditional recipes don't dilute the vinegar, but they are a bit too strong for my taste. You can also can the leaves using the water bath method (see "Water Bath Canning," page 236).

SOW THISTLE CAPERS

I love capers. I'll admit that these sow thistle capers can't replace the real thing, but I think it's quite cool that you can make an interesting caper substitute with wild stuff. If I recall correctly, we call them "poor man's capers" in Belgium, and yes, they're definitely cheaper.

Sow thistle is a plant native to Eurasia and Africa, but presently you will find it pretty much anywhere in the temperate regions of the world. In North America, the plant is considered a noxious weed or invasive in some areas.

You can create all kinds of "wild capers" with foraged ingredients, but one of the main denominators is the need for a very flavorful pickling solution. I don't think you can achieve the exact same flavor as true capers, but you can definitely make yours taste good or even great.

Personally, I stopped trying to duplicate the flavor of commercial capers long ago, and instead opted to embrace the possibilities that nature gifts me.

For sow thistle flower buds, you want to pick the rounded ones, which are the young and unopened flowers. The pointy buds come after the flowers bloom and the contents is mostly fluff—not usable for capers.

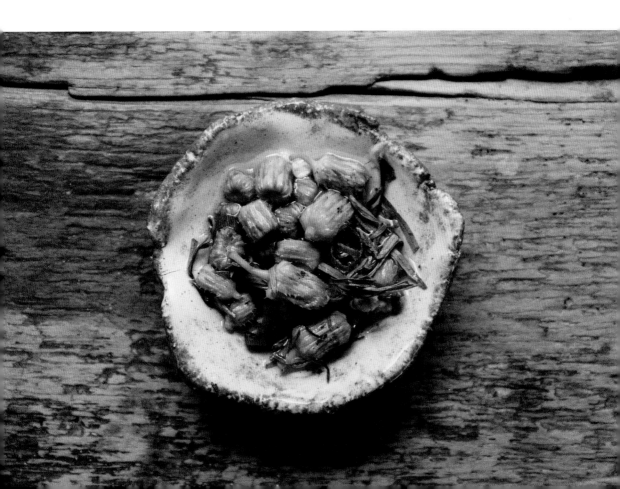

A typical caper-pickling solution is very salty. I normally use the following as a base:

1 tablespoon (15 ml) water (or white wine, beer)
3 tablespoons (45ml) vinegar of your choice
½ teaspoon (2.5 ml) maple syrup, honey, or 2 g sugar
¾ teaspoon (3.5 g) salt

Taste and adjust. Yes, it will be too salty, but realize that "capers" are really used for bursts of flavor in a dish.

You should also know that sow thistle buds are quite boring in terms of taste, so we need to add some zing to them. The vinegar you use is important, but so are the flavoring ingredients. If you sample a caper, you'll notice there is also some bitterness. It reminds me a bit of tarragon. Lucky for me, we have some wild tarragon locally, which I add to my pickling solutions for this recipe. I like a spicy kick too, and some sliced Thai chili does the work. A small amount of freshly grated ginger takes it to the next level.

Aside from the basic pickling solution, I've kept this recipe very vague on purpose, because it's really up to you to create the flavor profile and have fun. You could use Italian herbs, a za'atar blend, peppercorns, a touch of curry, or some ginger—you name it. Some people even use regular pickling spices, which are available in stores. Fermentation can really add an extra kick to your capers. A couple of years ago I added some sow thistle buds to a kimchi-type ferment for a couple of weeks, then quick pickled them. They were delicious.

There are tons of recipes online, too. Experiment, create *your* capers, and impress your guests.

Most of the time I just make a quick raw pickle using this basic recipe. It will easily keep for 2 to 3 weeks in the fridge. You can also use the water bath canning method for longer shelf life (see "Water Bath Canning," page 236).

For canning, simply bring the water, vinegar, maple syrup, and salt to a boil. Stir to make sure the salt is dissolved.

Place the sow thistle capers into the jar with the spices you are using, then pour the pickling solution over the top. Leave ½ inch (1.3 cm) headspace.

Screw on the lid, place in your water bath canner, and process for 12 minutes.

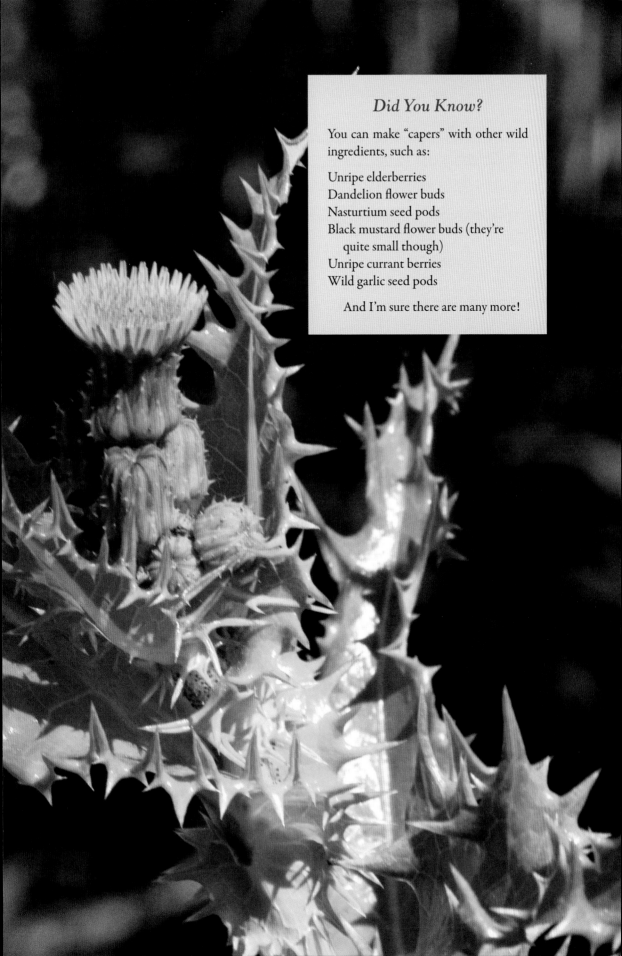

Did You Know?

You can make "capers" with other wild ingredients, such as:

Unripe elderberries
Dandelion flower buds
Nasturtium seed pods
Black mustard flower buds (they're
  quite small though)
Unripe currant berries
Wild garlic seed pods

And I'm sure there are many more!

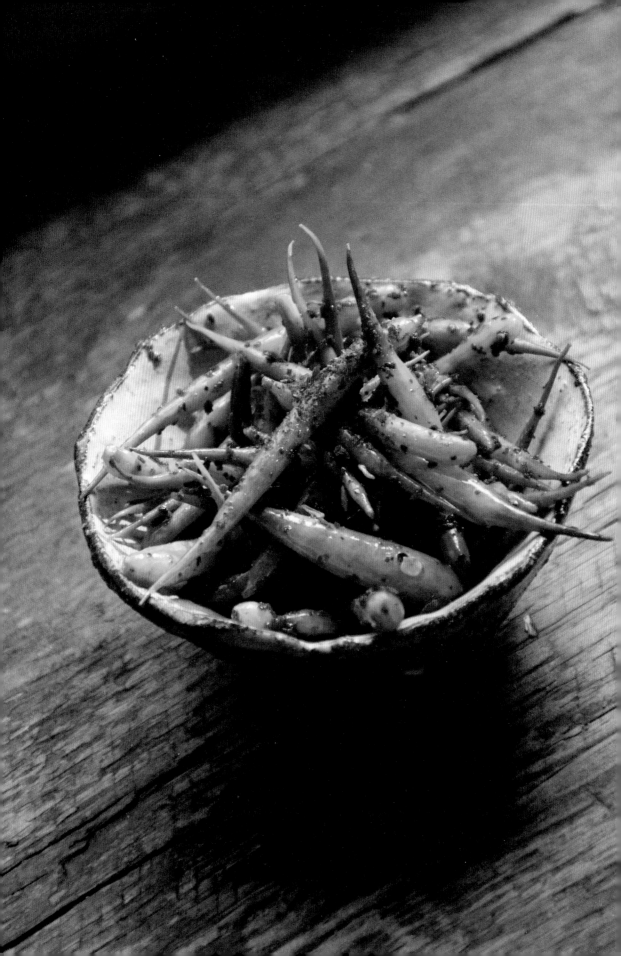

QUICK-PICKLED WILD RADISH PODS

Wild radish is one of the most common edible "weeds" I used to find locally in the Sylmar and Pasadena areas of Los Angeles. I think this quick pickle recipe would work with a variety of other wild edibles, such as sliced cattail shoots or burdock roots.

Every single part of the wild radish plant has culinary uses, from the tender root to the stem, leaves, seed pods, and flowers. My favorite parts are the pods. Foraging them is really about timing—you want to collect them while they're still juicy and flexible. At that stage they're delicious and taste better than the regular radishes you purchase at the store.

This recipe works very well with store-bought seasoned rice vinegar, but I like to use unpasteurized apple cider vinegar or homemade Apple Scraps Vinegar.

Ingredients for a small side dish for 2 people

1.4 ounces (40 g) radish pods
½ teaspoon (2.5 g) salt
3 tablespoons (45 ml) vinegar
2 teaspoons (10 ml) maple syrup or honey
1 tablespoon (15 ml) water or apple juice
1 teaspoon (2 g) chili flakes
½ teaspoon (1 g) grated fresh ginger

Procedure

Combine the radish pods and salt in a bowl and gently massage with your fingers for a minute or so, then let them rest for 15 to 20 minutes. The pods will become much more tender and juicy. Add the remaining ingredients. Ready to eat!

This quick pickle keeps in the fridge for 3 to 4 days, but the texture becomes too soft after that.

Note: *You can really get creative with this very basic recipe. I recently made a tasty version that included minced chervil and chickweed with a touch of ginger and garlic.*

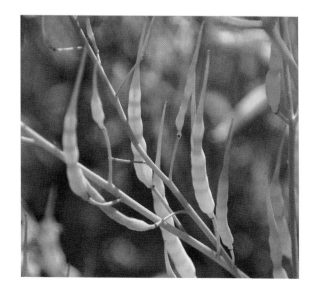

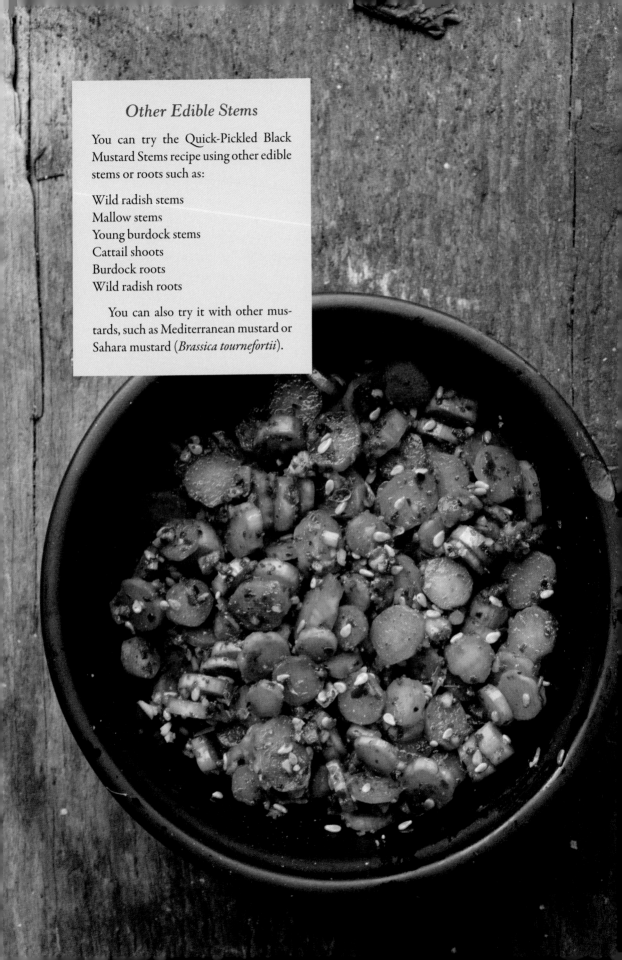

Other Edible Stems

You can try the Quick-Pickled Black Mustard Stems recipe using other edible stems or roots such as:

Wild radish stems
Mallow stems
Young burdock stems
Cattail shoots
Burdock roots
Wild radish roots

You can also try it with other mustards, such as Mediterranean mustard or Sahara mustard (*Brassica tournefortii*).

QUICK-PICKLED
BLACK MUSTARD STEMS

As I worked on this book, I found it interesting that some of my inspirations came from my last book, *Wildcrafted Fermentation*. Quite a few of the recipes, techniques, and culinary approaches therein can easily be adapted for quick pickles.

Pickled mustard stems are a good example. Minus the extra salt that is used for the lacto-fermentation, it's a good recipe for making a quick pickle. The result is a fantastic little side dish.

Black mustard leaves and flowers are spicy, with wasabi qualities, but the stems are quite sweet. They're a bit stringy, and the key is to slice them quite thin to break the fibers. Forage the mustard stems when they are still tender—usually late spring in Southern California.

I have prepared similar side dishes with tender mallow stems and burdock roots.

Ingredients for 1 serving

4 ounces (120 g) mustard stems
2 teaspoons (10 ml) seasoned vinegar
　　(or rice vinegar, or Mugwort Beer Vinegar
　　for me)
1 teaspoon (2 g) coriander seeds,
　　coarsely ground
1 teaspoon (2 g) chili flakes (spicy or not)
1 teaspoon (2 g) toasted sesame seeds
½ garlic clove, minced
½ teaspoon (2.5 ml) toasted sesame oil
　　(optional)
¼ teaspoon (0.5 g) curry powder

Procedure

Clean and slice the stems. Mix all the ingredients together in a bowl and serve fresh, or age for a few hours. I will keep this dish in the fridge for a few days, but it becomes mushy with longer aging.

QUICK-PICKLED WILD RADISH ROOTS

Wild radish is originally from Europe, Asia, and North Africa but can now be found all over the world, often as an invasive plant. Every single part of the wild radish plant can be used. Interestingly, the leaves of wild radish are identical to domesticated radish leaves. Radish leaves are sometimes sold in Korean grocery stores for making kimchi (yeolmu-kimchi).

The roots of wild radish, albeit smaller, are like daikon. The key to foraging tender radish roots is to find the right location and soil. In a tough soil with stones and such, the roots are usually gnarled and stringy. In sandy, soft ground, the root will go straight down, have room to expand, and will stay tender. You need a young plant—when it's flowering it's usually too late and the root will be too fibrous.

Ingredients for a 1-pint jar (480 ml)

8 ounces (227 g) sliced radish roots
½ cup (120 ml) vinegar (I like to use Elderberry Wine Vinegar)
½ cup (120 ml) water
3 tablespoons (45ml) maple syrup, honey, or sugar
0.7 ounce (20 g) sliced ginger
2 teaspoons (10 g) salt

Procedure

Clean the roots thoroughly. If you want, you can peel off the skin using a knife or vegetable peeler. Cut the root into thick slices. I like slices that are around ¼ inch (0.6 cm) thick, as they stay quite crunchy even after a few days in the vinegar solution.

Place all the ingredients in a pint (480 ml) jar, close it, and shake well to dissolve the sugar and salt.

Store in the fridge and enjoy within a month or so. If you like a nice crunch, it's much better if you serve it within a week.

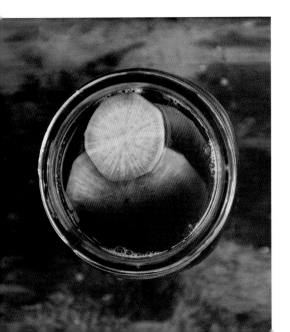

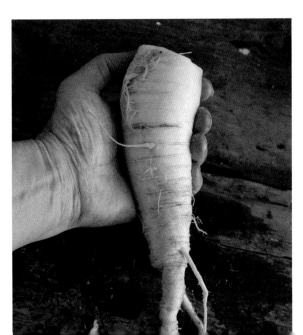

WILD RADISH ROOTS PICKLED IN FOREST BRINE

This is one of the most interesting quick pickles I've made. I think it's a great representation of how, through pickling, you can explore your local environment and the unique flavors it has to offer.

The vinegar is placed in a blender with local foraged herbs and made into a green, somewhat thick acidic liquid that is then used as the quick pickle solution. For the paste, I used wild chervil, chickweed, grass, miner's lettuce, filaree (*Erodium botrys*), and a bit of cilantro I had in the fridge.

You're not stuck with wild herbs; you can add all kinds of spices and other savory ingredients. In this case, I quick pickled some wild radish roots. But you can quick pickle anything—burdock roots, cucumbers, and so on. The idea is to use somewhat neutral ingredients that will benefit from the added green flavors of the pickling solution.

Ingredients for a 1-quart jar (1 L)

½ cup (120 ml) raw apple cider vinegar

¼ cup (60 ml) water or white wine

1 ounce (28 g) minced wild greens, mostly chickweed and chervil

0.5 ounce (14 g) minced cilantro

1.4 ounces (40 g) chopped green jalapeño

2 tablespoons (30 ml) maple syrup, honey, or brown or white sugar

0.7 ounce (20 g) chopped red onion

1 tablespoon (6 g) grated fresh ginger

½ teaspoon (2.5 g) sea salt

1½ to 2 cups (180 to 240 g) sliced wild radish root or cucumber

Procedure

Place all the ingredients except the radish roots in a blender and make a sort of liquid paste with the density of your choosing. As an alternative, you can use a molcajete. Either way, you end up with around 1½ cups (360 ml) of forest paste.

Place the wild radish roots in a quart (1 L) jar, add the paste, and age overnight in the fridge before serving.

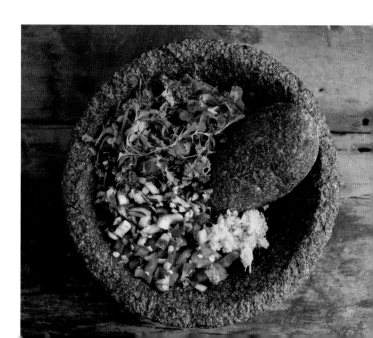

QUICK-PICKLED BURDOCK ROOT

Burdock is a plant native to Europe and Asia that has been introduced in pretty much every state in North America. It's non-native and considered invasive in many areas. Herbicides are recommended for removal, which of course is a bit silly when you realize that it's sold at Asian markets. Even my local supermarket carries it.

While the stalks are edible, my favorite part is the root. The flavor is incredibly earthy. You can stir-fry sliced roots with soy. My book *Wild-crafted Fermentation* features some delicious ferments with burdock roots, but even raw, they make for delicious pickles.

I don't want to compete too much with the root's flavor, so I keep the quick pickle recipe super simple. You can slice the roots as you would a carrot or make "french fries" with them (called batonnet cut)—either way works.

Ingredients for a 1-pint jar (480 ml)

Around 5 ounces (140 g) burdock roots, sliced

¾ cup (180 ml) unpasteurized apple cider vinegar or homemade Apple Scraps Vinegar

¼ cup (60ml) white wine (I use my white elderberry wine) or water or beer

2 tablespoons (30 ml) soy sauce

2 tablespoons (30 ml) maple syrup or sugar

0.5 ounces (14 g) ginger, sliced

2 spicy small chili pods (optional)

Procedure

Place the sliced burdock root into a jar, add all the other ingredients, then shake the contents well to dissolve the sugar.

Store in the fridge and wait a couple of days before consuming for optimum flavor. This quick pickle will keep for a month stored in the refrigerator.

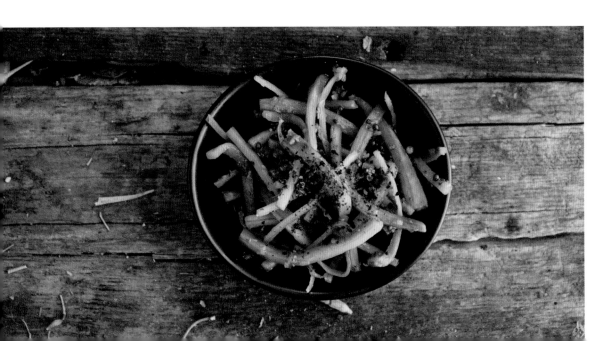

PICKLED RED ONIONS
IN FOREST HERBS

Not everything has to be wild. You can also take regular ingredients and infuse them with local plants for a unique, flavorful additive. I do this often with my most savory local wild herbs, such as fennel, chervil, wild mints, chickweed, mugwort, and others.

Some of the regular organic herbs that you can use are parsley, cilantro, and the like. Other vinegars of choice for this recipe include red Elderberry Wine Vinegar, Blackberry Wine Vinegar, and oak bark vinegar.

Ingredients for a
½-pint (240 ml) jar

2.5 ounces (70 g) red onions, sliced

4 tablespoons (60 ml) raw apple cider vinegar or homemade red wine vinegar

4 tablespoons (4.4 g) minced savory wild herbs (wild chervil, chickweed, and the like)

1 tablespoon (15 ml) water or white wine

2 teaspoons (30 ml) maple syrup

1 teaspoon (5 ml) olive oil (optional)

½ teaspoon (1 g) grated ginger or ginger powder

½ teaspoon (2.5 g) salt

¼ tsp (1 g) curry powder

Procedure

Place all ingredients in a bowl, and gently stir for a minute or so. Transfer the contents to the jar and screw the lid tight.

Store in the fridge and, for better flavor, wait a couple of days before consumption. This quick pickle will keep for around 10 days in the refrigerator.

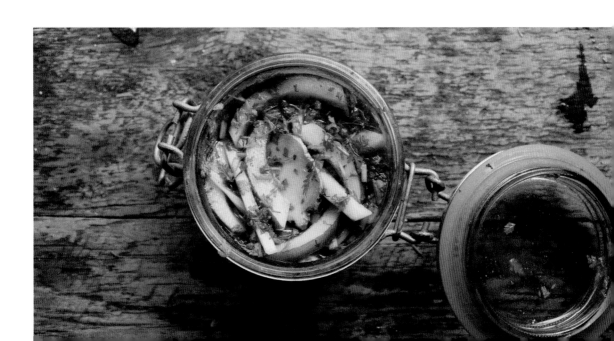

MUSHROOMS AND FOREST HERBS SALSA

You can create this salsa with commercial or wildcrafted mushrooms. The recipe is adaptable to your own environment. Think of it as a concept.

The inspiration for this recipe came from a local forest near Sylmar in Southern California. In early spring, oyster mushrooms are still quite abundant, and wild greens such as miner's lettuce, chickweed, chervil, and so on appear in good quantities. That makes this salsa a perfect representation of a specific place and moment in time. For this dish, I also use some bell peppers (red and orange) for aesthetic purposes.

Ingredients for around 10 ounces (280 g)

- 4.6 ounces (130 g) oyster or baby bella mushrooms or king boletes or chanterelles (or store-bought oyster or button mushrooms)
- 0.7 ounce (20 g) mixed savory wild greens (wild chervil, chickweed, and the like) or store-bought parsley or cilantro
- 2 tablespoons (30 ml) unpasteurized apple cider vinegar (I use Mugwort Beer Vinegar)
- 1 tablespoon (4 g) minced red chili pepper (spicy or not)
- 1 tablespoon (4 g) minced orange chili pepper (spicy or not)
- 1 tablespoon (15 ml) homemade or commercial stone-ground mustard
- 1 tablespoon (15 ml) maple syrup, honey, or sugar
- 0.5 ounce (14 g) minced green jalapeño
- 0.5 ounce (14 g) red onions, minced
- ½ teaspoon (1.5 g) dried thyme
- 1 Thai chili pepper, minced (optional)
- 1 garlic clove, minced
- 1 teaspoon (2 g) grated ginger
- ½ teaspoon (2.5 g) salt
- ¼ teaspoon (0.8 g) ground peppercorns
- 0.7 ounce (20 g) minced red and orange bell peppers

Procedure

Steam the mushrooms for around 15 minutes, or until they are well cooked. While the mushrooms are steaming, clean your wild greens and mince them.

After the mushrooms are steamed, let them cool off for a while, then mince them. In a bowl, combine all the ingredients and stir gently for a few seconds.

Place the bowl in the refrigerator and wait at least 30 minutes before serving. This will allow the flavors to blend.

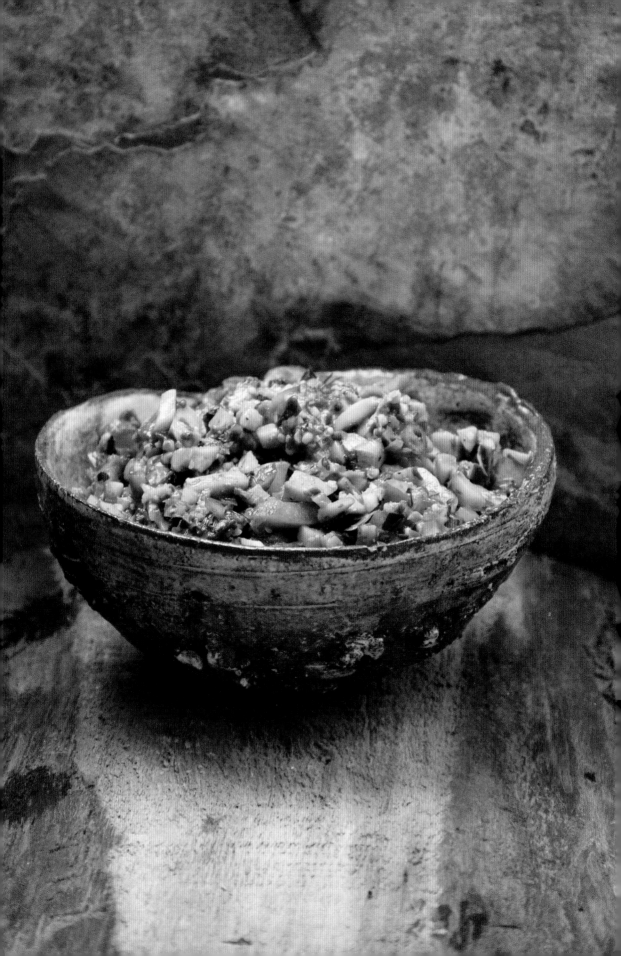

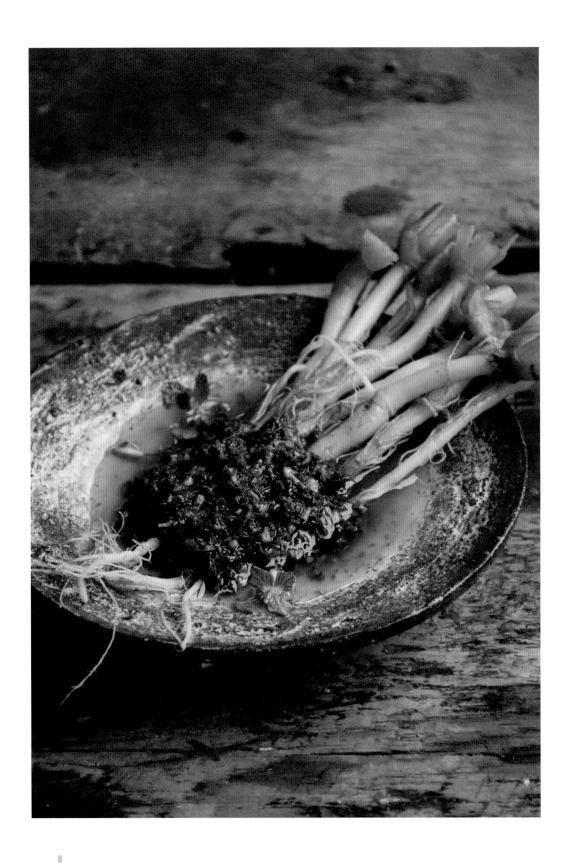

STEAMED WILD RADISH ROOTS, HERB OIL, AND SMOKED VINEGAR

This is somewhat of an odd dish, but it's so delicious. It's all about timing, as you must forage those roots at the right time.

I always say that wildcrafting is really about food preservation. This is a good example—you probably have a 2- to 3-week period to collect young radish roots. You can use them right away or you can freeze them. Lacto-fermentation would probably work too, but I like freezing these roots. That said, of course they're much better when you use them fresh.

The roots have a strong radish taste—eating more than 2 or 3 is a bit overwhelming. On the positive side, steaming them for 5 minutes will make them even more tender and reduce that piquant, spicy flavor.

I collected a bunch of chickweed and wild chervil while foraging my radish roots, then decided to make a dish based on that environment. The wild herbs are perfect for making a savory oil and vinegar dressing.

Ingredients to make
⅓ cup (80 ml) of herbs oil

1 cup (around 28 g) wild greens
  (chervil, chickweed, miner's lettuce,
  parsley, cilantro, or similar savory herbs)
2 medium garlic cloves
½ teaspoon (2.5 g) salt
¼ cup (60 ml) olive oil

Additional ingredients

8 to 10 tender radish roots
1 tablespoon (15 ml) unpasteurized
  apple cider vinegar or white wine vinegar
  or Mugwort Beer Vinegar

Procedure

Mince the greens and garlic cloves. Transfer the minced greens and garlic, salt, and olive oil into a blender. Process until you get the consistency you like, then set aside in a bowl.

Steam the young radish roots for 5 minutes.

Add the vinegar into the bowl containing the processed greens, garlic, and oil. A good apple cider vinegar or wine vinegar will work, but in this case, I used some of my Mugwort Beer Vinegar flavored with toasted oak bark that had been aged for a couple of years. Here is the advantage of using your own vinegar; you can't beat that flavor. But the dressing will still be awesome with a good unpasteurized apple cider vinegar.

Place the steamed roots on a plate and add the greens and vinegar oil on top. You're done!

By the way, you'll need bread with this. It's impossible not to eat the leftover oil and vinegar dressing.

BOILED LAMB'S-QUARTER AND
A DASH OF VINEGAR

This is pretty much boiled edible wild greens with a bit of seasoning. You can find similar humble dishes in many cultures.

In Greece, you'll find *horta*, which means weed or wild green. Horta is a generic name for a dish composed of wild edibles that are boiled or steamed, drained, then seasoned with olive oil, lemon juice, and spices. Korea has a similar dish called *namul*, in which the greens are boiled, drained, and often seasoned with fermented chili pepper paste, minced garlic, soy sauce, sesame oil, or other various condiments and spices.

In Belgium, my grandmother used to cook spinach, dandelion, and similar greens with fresh butter, milk, garlic, salt, and pepper.

My own version is similar to horta, but I use my own homemade vinegars instead of lemon juice. And I use young lamb's-quarter for this recipe. Stems may be too tough in older plants, but you can use the leaves.

Ingredients for one serving

3 ounces (85 g) young lamb's-quarter
  (stems and all) or watercress
  or other wild greens
2 teaspoons (10 ml) rice or raw
  apple cider vinegar (see Note)
1 teaspoon (5 ml) soy sauce (see Note)
½ teaspoon (1 g) grated ginger (optional)
1 small garlic clove, minced
¼ to ½ teaspoon (0.5–1 g) roasted
  sesame seeds
Salt and pepper, to taste

Procedure

Clean the lamb's-quarter.

Bring a pot of slightly salted water to a boil and cook the lamb's-quarter for a minute or so, then immediately transfer the greens into a bowl containing ice cold water.

When the lamb's-quarter is cold, drain the bowl. With clean hands, gently squeeze the lamb's-quarter to remove any excess water and transfer to a serving bowl.

In a separate small bowl, mix the vinegar, soy sauce, ginger, garlic, and sesame seeds. Pour the dressing over the cooked lamb's-quarter and mix well.

Taste and add salt or pepper if necessary.

Note: Infused vinegars, such as my Mountains Vinegar or seaweed vinegars (Seaweed-Infused Vinegar or Smoked Mushrooms and Seaweed–Infused Vinegar), will work well with this recipe. And as an alternative to soy sauce, you can use seasoned vinegar following my usual formula: 4 tablespoons vinegar to 2 teaspoons maple syrup to 1 teaspoon salt.

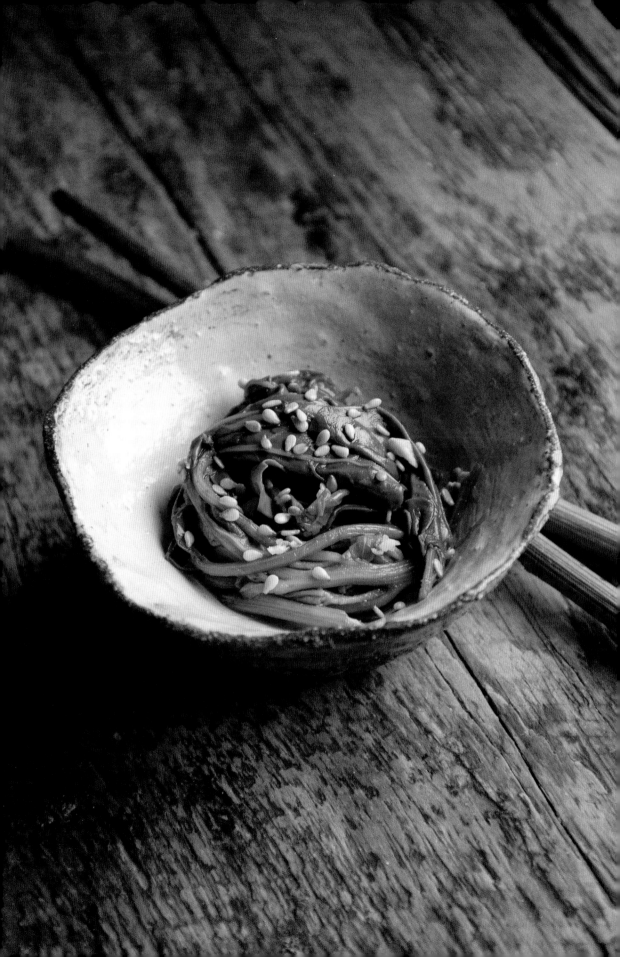

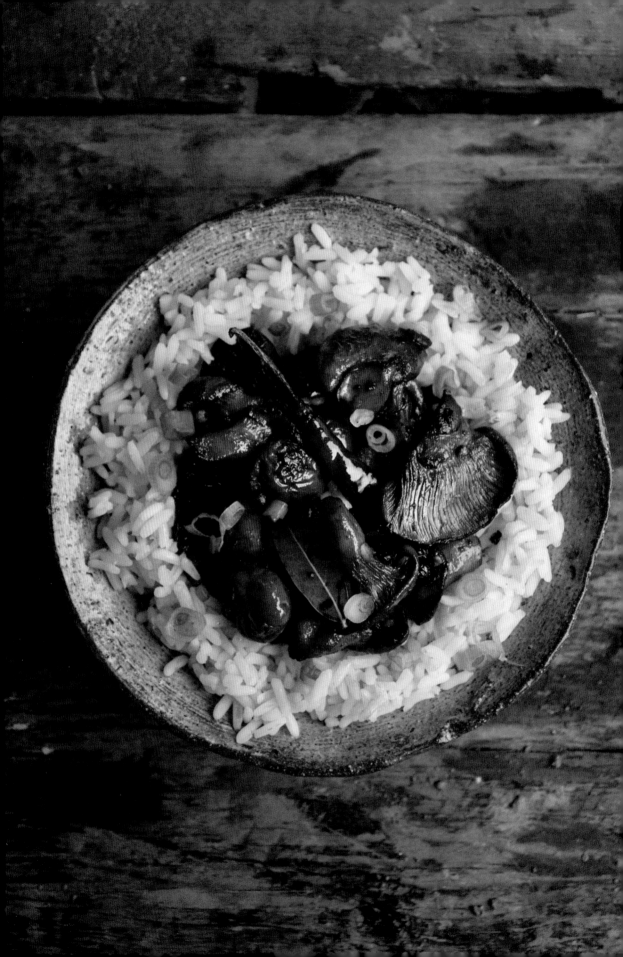

WILD OYSTER MUSHROOMS ADOBO

Adobo, or *adobar*, is a marinade of raw food (meat) in a vinegar solution with spices. Traditionally, this was a food preservation technique to allow meat to keep longer, but in modern times adobo is mostly known as a method of cooking meat with vinegar and spices. You'll find all kinds of variations on that concept in cultures and countries around the world. For example, the base of the Spanish (Iberian) version is usually composed of paprika, oregano, garlic, salt, and vinegar.

For this recipe, I cook wild oyster mushrooms instead of meat. Of course, you can use store-bought oyster mushrooms or substitute other edible wild or commercial mushrooms, including shiitake and crimini. This dish is best served with white rice and a touch of green onion. It's a tasty dish: sour, spicy, sweet, tangy.

Ingredients for 2 servings

8 ounces (240 g) baby oyster mushrooms
⅓ cup (80 ml) olive oil
⅓ cup (80 ml) red wine vinegar
    (I use Elderberry Wine Vinegar)
3 garlic cloves, ground to a paste
2 dried chili pods (optional)
1 teaspoon (1 g) dried oregano
    or a small sprig
1 teaspoon (2.5 g) paprika powder
1 teaspoon (5 ml) maple syrup
½ California bay leaf or 1 regular bay leaf
½ teaspoon (1 g) chili flakes (hot or not)
½ teaspoon (2 g) coriander seeds
Salt to taste

Some optional local (wild) flavors:

Around 6 Cracked Mediterranean-Style
    Green Olives (or store-bought
    green olives)
3 pieces (2 inches [5 cm] each) of
    California sagebrush stems
1 teaspoon (2 g) dried elderberries

Procedure

Mix all the ingredients, including any optional flavors, together in a bowl and transfer to a pan or small pot. I use a medium cast-iron pan. Cover the pan and cook at high heat for 10 minutes, then remove the lid and simmer for another 10 minutes. Make sure to stir from time to time.

Let most of the liquid evaporate, but not everything. If you want, you can save some of the sauce from earlier in the process and reduce it separately so you can control the texture and thickness of the dish.

WILD GRAINS SALAD

After summer, the landscape in many southern states on the West Coast is covered with dried-up vegetation, especially in Southern California. Most people assume there isn't anything to forage, but it's just an appearance. In reality we have a large number of edible grains and seeds that can be collected during this season and used in countless culinary applications. In the Los Angeles area, the local hills are covered with wild oats, cheatgrass, and wild barley.

The cool thing is that most of those grains are non-native and highly invasive, so eating them is helping the environment.

My inspiration for this dish came from one of my favorite Middle Eastern dishes, called tabbouleh. Tabbouleh is a vegetarian salad made with bulgur grain, minced parsley, and chopped onion, cucumber, and tomatoes. It is seasoned with lemon juice, olive oil, garlic, salt, and pepper. You'll find all kinds of variations in the recipe—some even use quinoa (*Chenopodium quino*) instead of bulgur grain.

Instead of parsley, I use local wild greens such as chickweed, wood sorrel, bur chervil, miner's lettuce, and the like.

Ingredients for 2 servings

1.7 ounces (45 g) wild oats and barley grains or commercial grains

½ teaspoon (2 g) cheatgrass grains (optional)

3 tablespoons (5 g) minced wild greens

1 tablespoon (7 g) chopped cucumber

1 tablespoon (7 g) chopped red onion

1 tablespoon (7 g) chopped red bell pepper

1 tablespoon (13 g) chopped tomato

2 teaspoons (.8 g) chopped green onions

2 tablespoons (30 ml) homemade Apple Scraps Vinegar, white wine vinegar, or rice vinegar

Salt and pepper to taste

½ garlic clove, minced (optional)

Procedure

Boil the wild oats and barley grains until chewy and tender (it usually takes around 20 minutes) then strain and set aside

Boil the cheatgrass grains for 50 minutes, then strain and remove the grains from the husk by hand. It may be tedious to do this, but cheatgrass provides a beautiful red grain that looks like rice. As an alternative, I often boil a large quantity of cheatgrass grains and freeze them after straining. You can thaw the frozen grains, remove the husk, and use them.

In a bowl, combine the cooked grains, wild greens, and chopped ingredients. Add the vinegar and mix gently. Add salt and pepper to taste.

I must say that this wild grains salad is absolutely delicious, very nutritious, and has earthy flavors that would be impossible to re-create using store-bought ingredients.

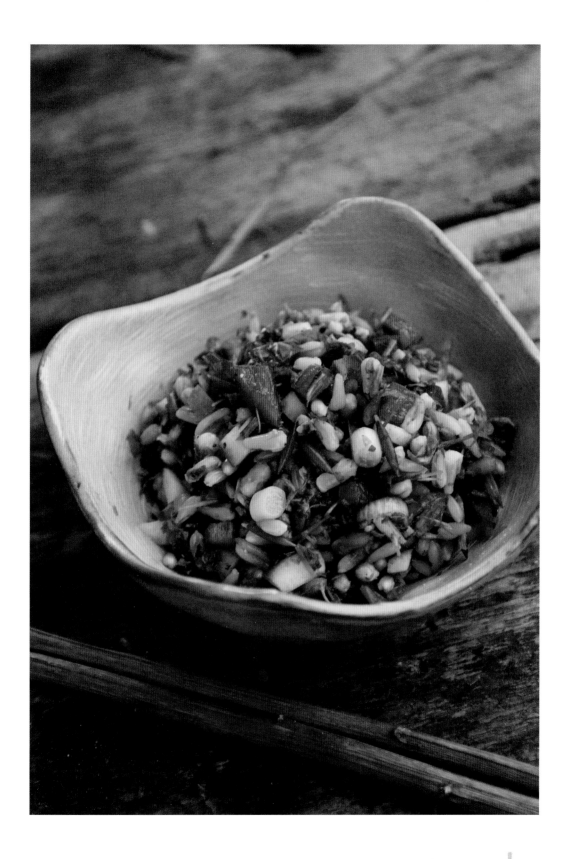

Wildcrafted Appetizers and Side Dishes | 215

STEAMED CRAYFISH

Some animals can be native in one state and invaders in another. The rusty crayfish (*Orconectes rusticus*), a native elsewhere, is an "invader" in Minnesota. We had a similar issue in Southern California with a different species of crayfish, but the problem with eating ours is the Los Angeles pollution. In Minnesota, the streams I found were pure, and so the crayfish were fine to eat.

For this dish, I use a special wild spice blend made from Southern California herbs that I used to grow in my native plants garden. I've perfected the recipe over the years. The flavor reminds me a bit of Old Bay Seasoning, although it's quite different in composition. It works perfectly for this dish.

You'll need to set your scale to grams to make this blend. You probably won't use everything so save some for next time.

Ingredients for ¾ cup (83 g) wild spice blend

6 grams whole peppercorns
4 grams white sage
3 grams California sagebrush
6 grams black sage
2 grams California bay leaf
32 grams garlic powder
30 grams coarse salt

Ingredients for two servings of crayfish

1 pound (455 g) cooked crayfish
3 tablespoons (45 ml) apple cider vinegar,
    Mugwort Beer Vinegar, or smoked
    Seaweed-Infused Vinegar
1 tablespoon (15 ml) water
1 tablespoon (6.8 g) wild spice blend
    or Old Bay Seasoning
2 to 3 teaspoons (5 to 7 g) chipotle powder

Procedure

Using a stone grinder or blender (like a Vitamix or electric coffee grinder), reduce the wild spice blend ingredients to a crude powder.

You can purchase cooked crayfish at the store, but if you collect them yourself, simply steam them for 5 minutes using a stainless-steel steamer basket.

Meanwhile, combine the vinegar, water, wild spice blend, and chipotle powder in a medium bowl.

Add the steamed crayfish into the bowl and gently mix the contents.

Place the bowl in the fridge to marinate for 3 to 4 hours, stirring the contents for a few seconds every hour or so, then serve.

Note: Instead of marinating the crayfish, another way to eat them is to make a sauce with the vinegar, water, and spices, then dip the tail meat in it while they are still hot.

WILD ONIONS IN VINAIGRETTE

This is a somewhat classic French dish usually made with commercial leeks, but the recipe is completely adaptable to wild garlic, leeks, and cattail shoots. You could also use green onions (scallions). I sometimes get a bit confused between wild onions, garlic, and leeks, but they're all from the same genus (*Allium*). Ramps, ramsons, or wild leeks are really types of wild onion.

Fresh onions are preferred for this recipe, but I've also used frozen wild onions. Here is what you need to make this simple and delicious dish.

Ingredients for 2 servings

12 small wild onions, commercial leeks, cattail shoots, or green onions (scallions)
4 cups (1 L) water
1 teaspoon (5 g) salt

Ingredients for ¼ cup (60 ml) of vinaigrette

1 teaspoon (5 g) Pickled Wild Seeds
2 teaspoons (6 g) minced red onion
½ garlic clove, minced
½ teaspoon (2.5 ml) maple syrup
2 teaspoons (10 ml) Stone-Ground Wild Black Mustard or store-bought Dijon mustard
1 tablespoon (15 ml) homemade red wine vinegar (see Note)
1 tablespoon (15 ml) olive oil
Salt and pepper to taste
½ teaspoon (1.5 g) dried wild (or commercial) tarragon

Procedure

Clean the wild onions to remove any dirt, then cut off the roots and the darker green tops. If you're using cattail shoots, you may need to remove some of the tougher skin layers.

Fill a sauce pot with the water, add the salt, and bring to a boil. Place the wild onions in the water and bring the contents to a brisk simmer for 7 to 8 minutes. For larger cattail shoots or ramps you may need to simmer for 10 minutes or so. Large commercial leeks may take up to 15 minutes.

Remove the wild onions, place on a paper towel, and let them cool.

In a bowl, mix the Pickled Wild Seeds, red onion, garlic, maple syrup, mustard, and vinegar. Whisk in the olive oil. Add salt and pepper to taste.

Place the cooked wild onions on a plate. Drizzle the vinaigrette and sprinkle the wild tarragon over them. Garnish with pickled wild radish pods and cured feral olives.

Note: Use any good-quality, fruity wine vinegar, such as blackberry, elderberry, or wild currant. They all work well for this recipe.

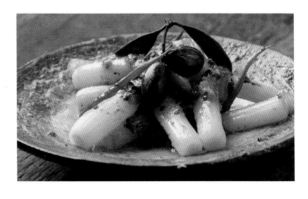

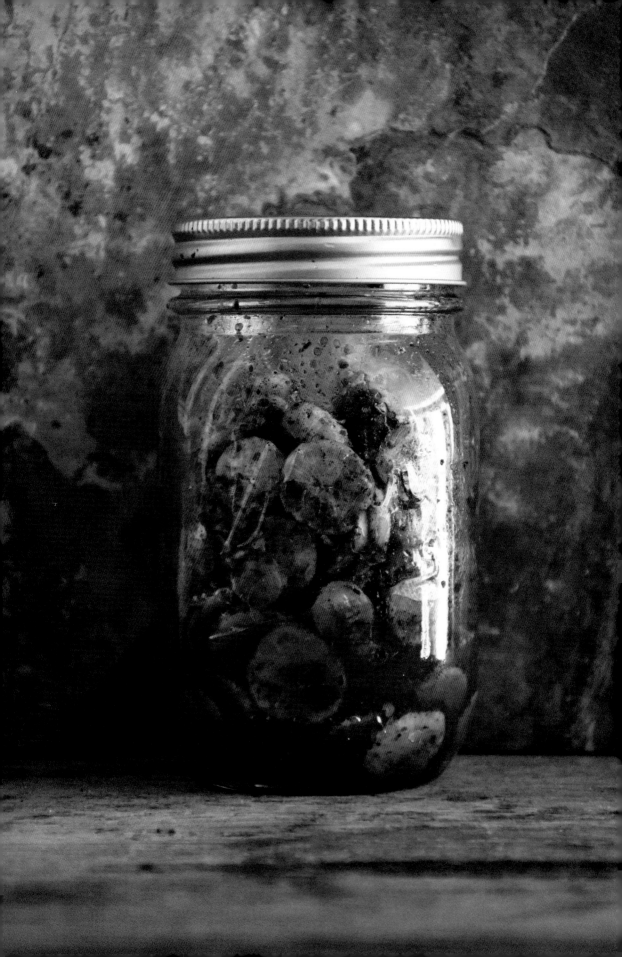

Fermented Plants with Vinegar

I call this process a double fermentation, but it's really a triple fermentation if you made your own alcoholic drink with which to create the vinegar. If you think about it, with a triple fermentation you're actually using every type of wild bacteria in North America or Europe that can be found in nature and used for fermentation: wild yeast, *Acetobacter*, and lactobacteria.

In short, you make the wine, beer, mead, or similar concoction with wildcrafted ingredients, then you turn it into vinegar naturally, and then you lacto-ferment some local wild food and use that vinegar to flavor it. You could not possibly find something like that commercially—it takes a deep personal connection with the environment and its microbiome to create it.

But you don't have to go all in with a triple fermentation to create delicious foods. You can take a shortcut by making a simple lacto-ferment, such as kimchi or sauerkraut, and adding a dash of seasoned vinegar when you serve it. The addition of savory seasoned vinegar to lacto-ferments was well received in the restaurants I worked with and in my wild food tasting workshops.

I have a whole book dedicated to the lacto-fermentation of wild edibles, called *Wildcrafted Fermentation*, if you want to go deeper into this subject. For now, we'll simply follow a specific recipe. And if you are an experienced fermenter, you already know what to do!

Lactobacteria exist on a lot of plants, including roots and vegetables, that have a decent amount of sugar. The secret of lacto-fermentation is rather simple: Bad bacteria that can spoil your food don't like salt, but lactobacteria don't mind it. Mixing salt with the ingredients you want to use will kill a lot of the bad bacteria and also draw the juice and sugar out of the ingredients through osmosis.

The lactobacteria convert the sugar to lactic acid, which creates an environment too acidic for the bacteria that can spoil your food. The high acidity is why lacto-ferments like sauerkraut or kimchi taste sour. The same principles apply to vinegar—a highly acidic environment helps with food preservation.

FERMENTED BURDOCK ROOTS
WITH SEASONED VINEGAR

Burdock roots are perfect for lacto-fermentation. Not only do they have a wonderful earthy flavor, but they contain a decent amount of sugar, which will be the main food source for the lactobacteria. You don't need anything special to make this ferment, nature will do the work.

You'll need some seasoned vinegar for this side dish. The sweetness will beautifully balance the ferment. You can use store-bought seasoned rice vinegar, or you can make your own by adding sugar and salt as indicated in this recipe.

Ingredients for a 1-pint jar (480 ml)

7 ounces (200 g) burdock roots
½ cup (120 ml) water for the brine
2 teaspoons (5 g) wild sumac powder
    (lemonade berries) or commercial
    sumac spice
2 teaspoons (4 g) dried lime powder,
    or loomi (optional)
2 teaspoons (5 g) mild chili powder
    (I use Korean chili flakes)
1 garlic clove, minced
A bit more than 1 teaspoon of salt (6 g)
1 teaspoon (2 g) grated ginger
½ teaspoon (1.5 g) smoked jalapeño powder

Ingredients for slightly more than ¼ cup (60 ml) of seasoned vinegar

4 tablespoons (60 ml) vinegar
2 teaspoons (10 ml) maple syrup or honey
½ teaspoon (2.5 g) salt

Lacto-Fermentation Procedure

Clean the roots in cold water. Be gentle—I normally use a sponge, which helps remove the dirt. The lactobacteria are present on the skin, so don't peel it off.

Slice the roots and place them into a bowl of cold water immediately so they don't turn brown. Transfer the roots to another bowl and add all the other main ingredients. Massage gently for a minute, then let everything rest for 10 minutes. Massage one more time and place in the jar. Close the lid.

The ingredients won't be covered by the brine, so you'll need to shake the contents 2 to 3 times a day to distribute the acidity as fermentation takes hold. Sometimes I even place the jar upside down for a few hours. Burp as necessary.

Ferment for 10 to 15 days, or until you get no more fermentation gases, then place the jar in the fridge. You can keep this ferment in the fridge for well over 6 months.

Quick Pickle Procedure

To make a side dish for 2 people, I simply remove around 1.5 to 2 ounces (43 to 56 g) of fermented burdock slices from the jar, place them in a small bowl, and add 2 to 3 teaspoons (10 to 15 ml) of seasoned vinegar.

Mix gently with a fork or your (clean) fingers and wait at least 15 minutes before serving. You can add fresh herbs if you want. This dish is quite delicious; earthy, salty, spicy, sweet . . . all the good stuff in a small serving bowl.

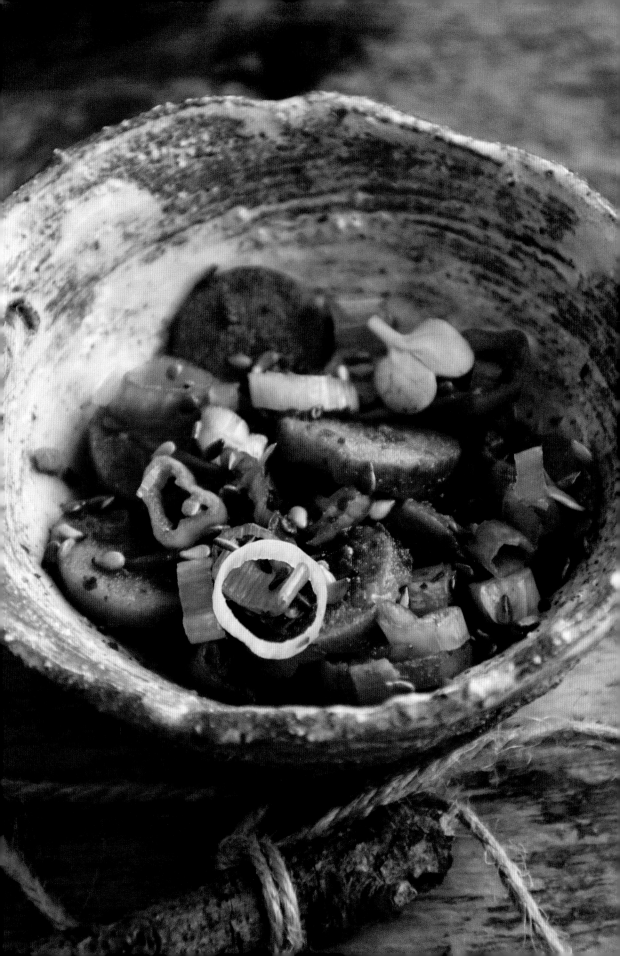

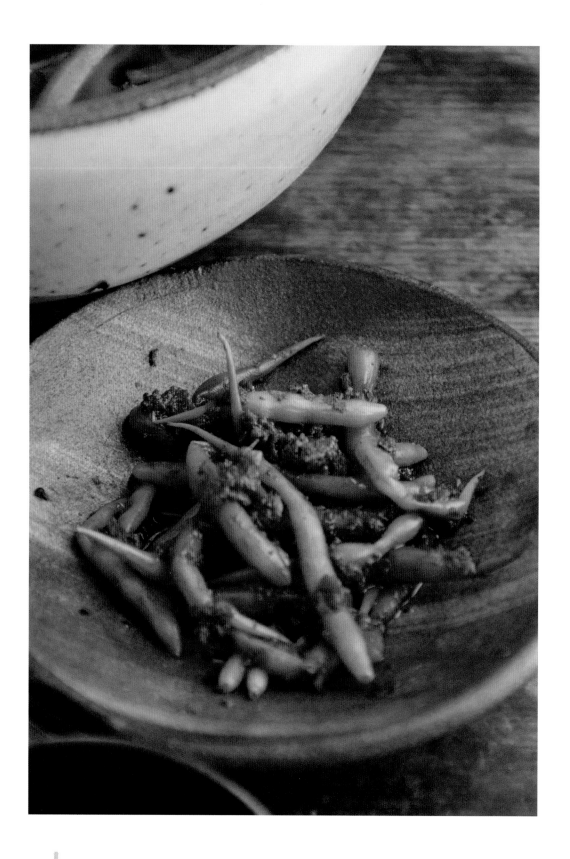

FERMENTED RADISH PODS WITH SEASONED VINEGAR

This dish is easy to make and it's fantastic as a side dish or as an addition to salads or sandwiches. The method is very similar to that for the fermented burdock roots. You can even use the same spices, but in this case I use a homemade barbecue spice blend.

Ingredients for 3 tablespoons (20 g) of barbecue spice blend

1 tablespoon (9 g) smoked paprika powder
1 teaspoon (3 g) smoked chipotle powder
1 teaspoon (4.5 g) brown sugar
½ teaspoon (1.5 g) ground peppercorn
½ teaspoon (1.5 g) garlic granules or powder
½ teaspoon (1.5 g) onion powder
½ teaspoon (1.5 g) ginger powder

Ingredients for a ½-pint jar (240 ml) of fermented radish pods

7 ounces (200 g) wild radish pods
1 teaspoon (5 g) salt
2 cloves garlic, finely chopped
0.7 ounces (20 g) barbecue spice blend
¼ cup (60 ml) water

Pickling ingredients for 2 servings

1 ounce (28 g) fermented radish pods
2 teaspoons (10 ml) seasoned unpasteurized apple cider vinegar (see previous recipe)

Lacto-Fermentation procedure

Mix the wild radish pods, salt, and garlic and massage tenderly for 2 to 3 minutes. Let everything rest for 20 minutes, then massage it again and let it rest again for 15 minutes. You want the salt to start extracting moisture. The mix should be quite wet and the pods soft and tender. This makes it easier to pack them in the jar. Meanwhile, mix the spice blend ingredients together to make the barbecue blend.

When the pods are ready, add the barbecue spice blend and massage again for 2 to 3 minutes, then pack everything into the jar. No need to pack too tightly. Finally, add the water.

The ingredients won't be covered by the brine, so you'll need to shake the contents 2 to 3 times a day to distribute the acidity as fermentation takes hold. Sometimes I even place the jar upside down for a few hours. Burp as necessary.

Ferment for 10 to 15 days, or until you get no more fermentation gases, then place the jar in the fridge. You can keep this ferment in the fridge for well over 6 months.

Quick pickling procedure

Gently mix the radish pods and seasoned vinegar with a fork or your (clean) fingers and wait at least 15 minutes before serving.

SPICY WILD FERMENT
WITH SEASONED VINEGAR

This wild food ferment is composed of locally foraged black mustard and wild radish leaves fermented with chili flakes or chili powder and garlic. As I often do, I mix in some regular ingredients—bok choy and green cabbage. It's much better in terms of flavors and it ends up tasting more like a regular kimchi. You could use napa cabbage, too.

Because of seasonality, you can't really make the same recipe twice, so this is again a concept recipe. Every location provides different ingredients, too. If I'm in Colorado, for example, I use garlic mustard; whereas if I'm in Southern California, I use black mustard. You are looking at a ratio of around 30 percent wildcrafted ingredients to 70 percent regular stuff, but you can experiment and use a higher proportion of wild edibles.

Ingredients for a 1-quart jar (1 L) ferment

12 ounces (340 g) bok choy leaves

4 ounces (120 g) shredded green cabbage

1 tablespoon (15 g) salt

4 ounces (120 g) wild mustard and radish leaves or other wild greens

1 ounce (28 g) curly dock leaves

6 garlic cloves

⅓ cup (80 ml) water

2 to 4 tablespoons (10 to 20 g) mild chili flakes

1 teaspoon (2 g) spicy chili flakes (I use smoked jalapeño flakes)

Lacto-Fermentation Procedure

Place the bok choy and cabbage in a bowl, add the salt, and gently massage the ingredients for 10 minutes. Let the contents rest for 20 minutes, then repeat twice until the leaves are tender and you have a decent amount of brine. Don't massage the bok choy too hard the first time, as it may break the stems and leaves.

Meanwhile, cut all the wild greens and curly dock leaves in thin strips (chiffonade), mince the garlic, and get all the other ingredients ready.

Place all the ingredients into the bowl containing the bok choy and cabbage. Massage one more time for 3 to 4 minutes, this time wearing gloves to protect your hands from the chili flakes.

Transfer the contents into a jar to ferment for around 3 to 5 days at room temperature. Burp as necessary and stir the contents at least once a day with a clean fork. Once the fermentation is complete, store the jar in the fridge, where it will keep for weeks.

Note: Seasoned rice vinegar works fantastic with this dish, but your own homemade seasoned vinegar can be just as awesome. For my last wild food tasting, I used a seasoned smoked Seaweed-Infused Vinegar.

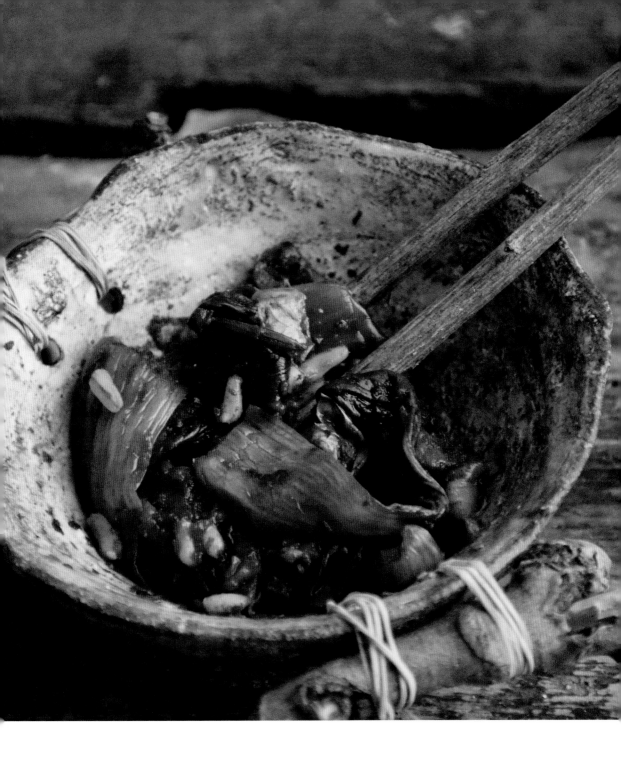

Ingredients for 2 servings as a side-dish

1.5 to 2 ounces (43 to 56 g) of ferment

2 to 3 teaspoons (10 to 15 ml)
seasoned vinegar (see Note)

Side-Dish Procedure

Mix the ferment and seasoned vinegar gently with a fork or your (clean) fingers, and wait at least 15 minutes before serving.

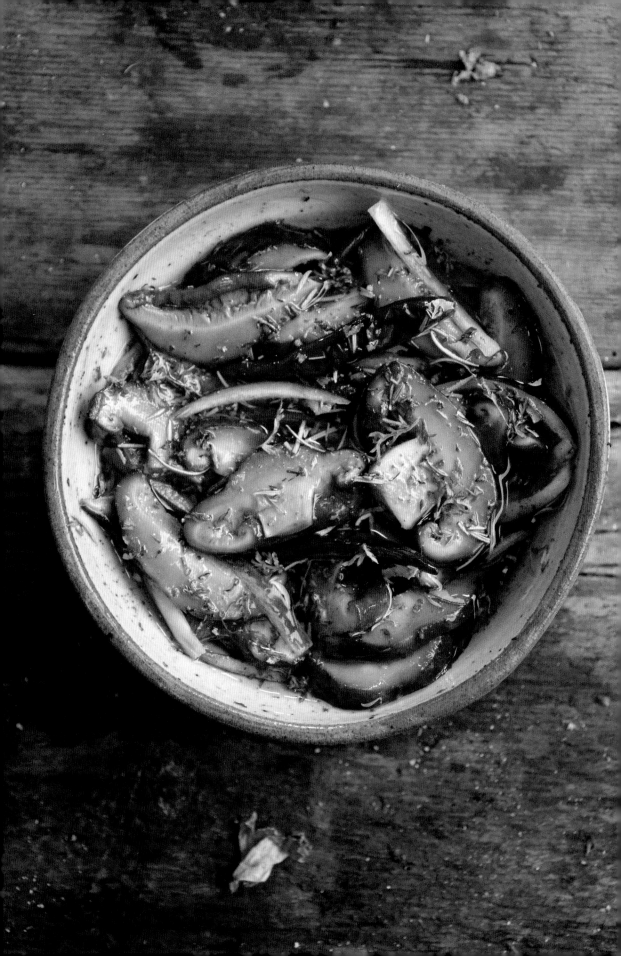

LACTO-FERMENTED SHIITAKE
IN VINEGAR

Lacto-fermented mushrooms are quite tasty, and quick pickling them with a good homemade vinegar and spices makes for a delicious side dish. As explained in my book *Wildcrafted Fermentation*, the key to success when fermenting mushrooms is the addition of a sugar source to feed the lacto-bacteria. In this recipe, instead of using salt I use soy sauce. The same procedure will work with other wild mushrooms, such as oysters, morels, pheasant's backs, and many more.

Ingredients for a
1-pint jar (480 ml) ferment

12 ounces (340 g) shiitake mushrooms

¾ cup (180 ml) water

3 tablespoons (45 ml) soy sauce

2 tablespoons (30 ml) sauerkraut juice
   or whey as a culture starter

1 tablespoon (15 ml) maple syrup,
   honey, or sugar

1 or 2 dehydrated chili pods (spicy or not)

2 garlic cloves, crushed

½ California bay leaf or 1 regular bay leaf

Ingredients for 2 servings
as a side dish

2.5 ounces (70 g) fermented mushrooms

¼ small red onion, sliced

2 teaspoons (10 ml) red wine vinegar
   (I use Elderberry Wine Vinegar)

2 teaspoons (10 ml) olive oil

1 teaspoon (5 ml) maple syrup

1 teaspoon (5 ml) stone-ground Dijon mustard

1 teaspoon (5 ml) water

¼ teaspoon (0.8 g) herbs blend
   (Italian herbs or herbes de Provence)

Lacto-Fermentation procedure for the ferment

Steam the mushrooms for 20 minutes. Wild mushrooms should always be cooked. Some, like morels, can be toxic when raw.

Combine all the ferment ingredients in the pint jar.

With the amount I purchased at my local Asian foods supermarket, I ended up with 12 ounces (340 g) of steamed mushrooms. Normally, I use 2 teaspoons (10 g) of salt for every pound (455 g) of ingredients I want to ferment. Following that rule, I would need to use 1½ teaspoons (7.5 g) of salt, but for this recipe I replaced salt with soy sauce. To do so, simply multiply the amount of salt by 6. Thus, I used 3 tablespoons (45 ml) of soy sauce.

The lactobacteria on the mushrooms will have been killed during steaming. The solution is to add the sauerkraut juice (or yogurt whey) as a culture starter and maple syrup to feed the bacteria.

Ferment for 10 to 15 days in a jar, shaking and burping at least twice daily. Once the fermentation is complete, store the jar in the fridge, where it will keep for at least 3 to 4 months.

Quick pickling procedure for the side dish

Gently mix the side dish ingredients with a fork or your (clean) fingers and wait at least 15 minutes before serving.

WILD OYSTER MUSHROOMS IN SEASONED VINEGAR

You can make this dish with fermented wild oyster mushrooms, but in this case, I just steamed them and skipped the fermentation process. Either way, it's a great side dish. My preference is to use small "baby" mushrooms, which are firmer.

For 1½ cup (360 ml) of seasoned vinegar

¾ cup (180 ml) homemade Apple Scraps Vinegar or store-bought unpasteurized apple cider vinegar
½ cup (120 ml) water
2½ tablespoons (37 ml) maple syrup
1½ teaspoons (7.5 g) salt

Ingredients for 2 servings

7 ounces (200 g) steamed or fermented oyster mushrooms
1¼ cup (300 ml) seasoned vinegar
3.5 ounces (100 g) red onions, sliced
2 wild pequin chili peppers (optional—you can also use regular chili flakes)
0.2 ounces (5 g) grated ginger
½ teaspoon (3 g) ground peppercorns
2 dill or wild chervil sprigs

Procedure

Mix together the seasoned vinegar ingredients and set aside.

If you're using raw (not fermented) mushrooms, steam them for 20 minutes. Mix all the ingredients together in a clean bowl, then store in the refrigerator for a few hours before eating.

Quick pickling procedure for the side dish

Gently mix the side dish ingredients with a fork or your (clean) fingers and wait at least 15 minutes before serving. You can store this for at least a week.

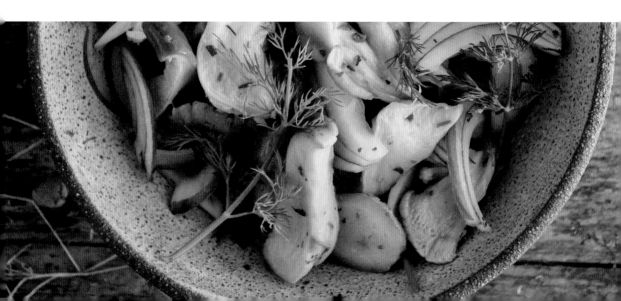

CHAPTER 7

Preserves, Soups, and Drinks

One of the main roles of vinegar is, of course, food preservation. As explained earlier in the book, the science behind the use of vinegar for food preservation is simple. Bacteria and mold that could spoil the food can't proliferate in an acidic environment. The acetic acid present in vinegar guarantees that your mushrooms, roots, or vegetables won't spoil.

In this chapter, we'll look at a few traditional preserves that don't require placing jars in boiling water to pasteurize the contents—such as pickled eggs, olives, or garlic heads—and we'll also look at a modern food preservation technique called water bath canning.

There are a lot of creative possibilities with canning and wild greens: You can make preserves that cannot be found in regular stores, such as pickled radish pods, cattails, walnuts, and so on. I think water bath canning is a fantastic method to explore for creating condiments that are a good representation of local flavors.

A whole book could be written on using this preservation method with wild edibles. I'm barely touching the subject in this chapter, but the few basic recipes and procedures featured here can be applied to other wild edibles. For example, you can use the same procedure for pickling wild radish pods with black mustard stems or unripe sow thistle flowers.

This chapter also features a few examples of soups that incorporate vinegar. I think you'll find them very useful with edible plants that have a bitter edge, such as mustard or radish greens, watercress, dandelion, thistle, and the like. In the old days it was not uncommon to add vinegar and sugar to soups in order to counteract the slight bitterness of the ingredients. My mom often added a splash of balsamic vinegar to the countless soups she would create to balance and enhance the flavors. Many traditional soups contain vinegar—French onion soups, mallow soup in the Middle East, hot and sour Chinese soup, and so on.

And finally, we'll explore some tasty and healthy wilder drinks that use vinegar as the main component. Some of them are quite similar to the popular kombucha drinks.

GARLIC HEADS PICKLED
IN ELDERBERRY WINE VINEGAR

Recipes for garlic preserved in vinegar and spices can be found in many cultures and countries, from the Middle East (*torshi seer*) to Thailand (*gratiem dong*) to China (*táng suàn*) and to Europe (though in Europe it's not very common anymore).

The choice of spices and vinegars varies immensely. As usual, I thought this kind of pickling would be perfect with the addition of local wild flavors. I use dried elderberries and California bay leaves, but, for example, in Iran, some recipes use dried barberries and local spices. My friend in Northern California uses huckleberries instead of elderberries.

Ingredients for a 1-quart jar (1 L)

1¼ cups (300 ml) red wine vinegar
   (I use Elderberry Wine Vinegar)
¼ cup (60 ml) balsamic vinegar
1½ tablespoons (23 ml) soy sauce
3 tablespoons (45 ml) maple syrup
1½ tablespoons (17 g) dehydrated elderberries
½ California bay leaf or 1 bay leaf
½ teaspoon (1.5 g) whole peppercorns
2 to 3 slices (6 g) fresh ginger
2 spicy chili pods
Enough garlic heads to loosely fill the jar
   (about 10 medium heads)

Procedure

Combine all the ingredients but the garlic in a small pot and bring the contents to a boil.

Meanwhile, remove most of the outer papery skins from your garlic heads and place them in a clean jar. Pour the boiling pickling solution over them and close the jar. Make sure the garlic heads stay submerged. (See Note.)

Store in a cool, dark place for at least 6 months, but it will get much better if you age it longer (one year or much more). *Torshi seer*, the similar Middle East ferment, can be aged for years.

> *Note: Despite pouring a boiling hot pickling solution in the jar, it's possible that your garlic heads will start fermenting after 3 to 4 days. If this is the case, you may need to release the fermentation gases by opening the lid briefly a couple of times a day. The fermentation part usually ends after a couple of weeks.*
>
> *Pickled garlic cloves can be served as a condiment or added to salad and soups. During the aging process, the garlic flavor and texture will change quite radically to something more tender, mellow, and fruity.*

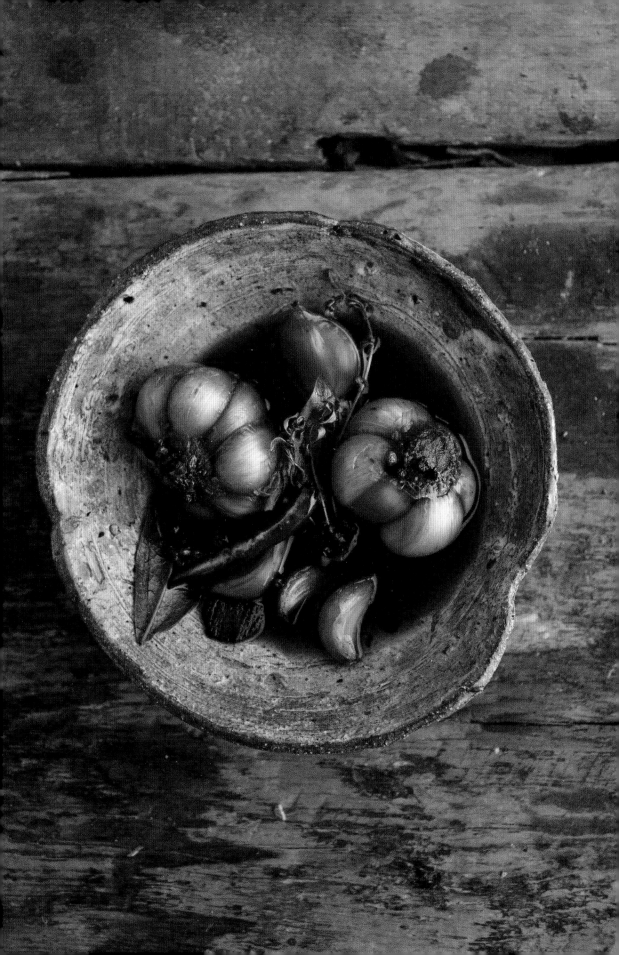

OYSTER MUSHROOM JERKY

During a wet winter, which is rare these days, there can be a real abundance of oyster mushrooms in the Los Angeles area. A couple of years ago, I found probably over 60 pounds (27 kg) of them, which was way too much to even contemplate collecting.

That said, I used a bunch of different methods to preserve the harvest, such as freezing, canning, dehydrating, and so on.

One of my favorite food preservation activities is making oyster mushroom jerky, which I love to share with my students. This recipe is vinegar-based and super tasty. The marinade is also a good fit for other wild or commercial mushrooms.

Ingredients for 2 servings

1 pound (455 g) large oyster mushrooms
½ cup (120 ml) vinegar (I use Mugwort Beer Vinegar, and apple cider vinegar will work great)
½ cup (120 ml) soy sauce (or Worcestershire or A.1. steak sauce)
2 tablespoons (30 ml) maple syrup or honey
1½ tablespoons (13 g) garlic powder
1 tablespoon (15 ml) sesame oil
1 tablespoon (9 g) onion powder or small shallot, diced
2 teaspoons (6 g) Italian herbs blend or herbes de Provence
2 teaspoons (4 g) chili flakes or powder
2 teaspoons (3.8 g) ground coriander seeds (optional)
1 teaspoon (3 g) curry powder (optional)
1 teaspoon (5 ml) liquid smoke (optional)
0.35 ounce (10 g) ginger, sliced (optional)
½ teaspoon (0.8 g) ground black pepper
½ California bay leaf or 1 regular bay leaf

Procedure

I use the largest mushrooms I've collected to make this jerky. The diameter will vary from 5 to 8 inches (12.5 to 20 cm). Slice the mushrooms thinly, around ¼ inch (0.6 cm) thick, and steam them for 20 minutes.

Meanwhile, in a large bowl, combine the rest of the ingredients to make the marinade. Let the mushroom slices cool off after steaming and place them into the marinade.

Stir the slices in the marinade for a minute or so, then cover the bowl with plastic wrap and place in the fridge for 8 to 12 hours.

Remove the mushroom slices from the marinade and lay them out on a baking tray. I set my oven to the lowest temperature (160°F, or 70°C) to dehydrate them. It takes slightly more than 8 hours. Another (faster) way to do it is to bake the mushrooms for around 2 hours at 230°F (110°C), making sure to turn the mushrooms after an hour of baking. You can sprinkle additional chili flakes on the marinated jerky prior to dehydration (see Note).

Enjoy, and keep the leftovers in an airtight container in the refrigerator.

Note: *You want to stop dehydrating them when you feel they're still pliable like regular jerky, unless you like to chew on super dry stuff.*

Feel free to create around this recipe and change up the ingredients.

PICKLED QUAIL EGGS
IN WILD BEER AND VINEGAR

I have a whole book dedicated to wild brews, called *The Wildcrafting Brewer*, but even if you don't make your own beers out of wild plants, you can use a good artisanal beer for this recipe.

Pickled quail eggs have been a classic for years in the wild food tasting menu I offer at the end of a foraging class.

Ingredients for a 1-quart jar (1 L)

20 quail eggs

1 cup (240 ml) unpasteurized
apple cider vinegar or red wine vinegar
(5 percent acidity)

½ cup (120 ml) homemade vinegar
(I use my Elderberry Wine Vinegar)

½ cup (120 ml) beer of your choice
(red wine would work, too)

½ cup (120 ml) water

2 tablespoons (30 ml) maple syrup,
honey, or sugar

1 tablespoon (15 g) salt

Just under 1 tablespoon (8 g) pickling spices
blend (store-bought)

1 tablespoon (6 g) dried elderberries
(optional)

½ California bay leaf or 1 bay leaf

1 garlic clove, crushed

1 teaspoon (2 g) chili flakes

Procedure

Place the quail eggs in a pot and cover with cold water. Bring the water to a boil, then immediately remove from the heat. Let the eggs stand in the hot water for 5 minutes, then transfer them into cold water. Once they are cool, carefully remove the shells.

In a pot, prepare the brine with the remaining ingredients. Bring the brine to a boil, then remove from heat.

Place the eggs in a clean jar, leaving 1 inch (2.5 cm) headspace, and fill the jar with the hot brine. Close the lid and refrigerate for a week before serving. They will keep in the fridge for at least a month.

The eggs will end up with a dark red color from the elderberries and wine vinegar.

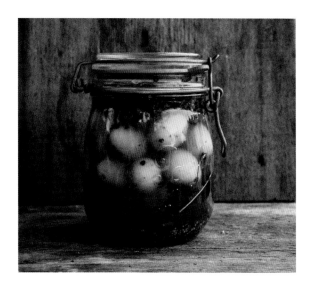

CRACKED MEDITERRANEAN-STYLE GREEN OLIVES

Not using local, plentiful wild food is truly a form of food waste. Such is the case with the countless feral olive trees that exist in the San Fernando Valley in Southern California. I lived there for 20 years and never saw anyone picking them. Thousands of pounds are going to waste every year.

I like to forage these olives (mission olives) while they're still green, but to make sure that they are "green-ripe," you need to test and squeeze a few. If they release a creamy white juice, they are ready to harvest. My favorite traditional way to preserve them is to make cracked green olives.

Fresh olives are naturally very bitter. To make them palatable, you must first cure them to remove a bitter chemical compound called oleuropein. Once this is done, they can be preserved in a vinegar and salt brine. Here is the method.

Ingredients for four to five 1-quart jars (4–5 L), depending on olive size

5 pounds (2.3 kg) green olives
¾ cup (180 g) salt
2 quarts (2 L) filtered water
1 cup (240 ml) vinegar
Herbs, spices, and other seasonings of your choice (optional), see step #6

Procedure

1. Clean your olives in cold water, removing any that are bruised or possibly infected with olive fly larvae. The infection is quite visible—you'll see obvious brown spots and a small indentation or lump on the surface of the fruit.
2. Take your cleaned olives and one by one, crack them open using a mallet or a stone.

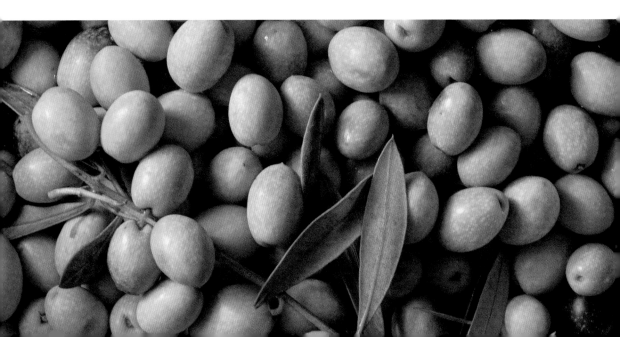

3. Place the cracked olives in a food grade bucket or glass container and cover them with water. You can use tap water for this part. I use a small plate to keep them under the surface of the water. Change the water daily.
4. Taste them after 5 days. If they're still too bitter, keep changing the water. You really go by taste on this process, but you don't want them to lose all their bitterness.
5. Make a brine with the salt, filtered water, and vinegar.
6. Drain the olives, place them in quart (1 L) jars, and cover them with the brine. Note that you can add herbs, spices, and other seasonings, as well. In each jar I usually add half of a lemon, sliced; one sprig of thyme; a couple of spicy chili pods; and 3 crushed garlic cloves. Commercial pickling spices would work well, too.
7. Place in the refrigerator and wait 2 to 3 weeks before eating them. They will keep for up to a year.

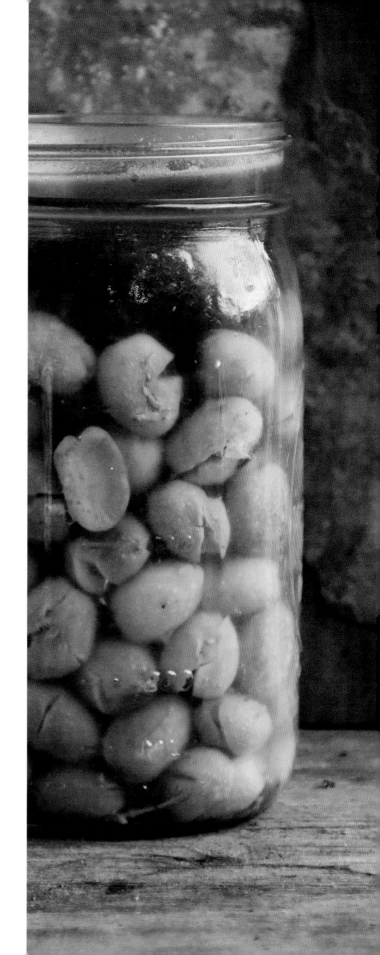

Water Bath Canning

The most used method for preserving acidic food in closed jars is called water bath canning. It's not a complicated process. The idea is to bring the jars to a temperature high enough to kill any living organism that could spoil the food (pasteurization). Such preserves can be stored at room temperature for at least a year. It is recommended that you use a vinegar with at least 5 percent acidity for recipes preserved using water bath canning.

For small batches, I often use a regular pot and a specifically designed mesh between the jars and the bottom of the pot, so the jars don't directly touch the hot surface. But if you are new to this, I strongly suggest you purchase a boiling water canner.

Tools you'll need:

> Canning jars, lids, and bands
> Thermometer
> Jar lifter
> Jar funnel
> Boiling water canner

The following procedure can be used for any of the recipes in this book, unless the recipe is intended to be raw or you are making a quick pickle.

1. Fill your canner with warm water. Depending on the size of the jars you will be using, adjust the amount of water so there will be couple of inches over the jars. Heat your water to around 140°F (60°C).
2. Fill your jars with your recipe, making sure to leave at least ½ inch (1.3 cm) headspace.
3. Place the lid on each jar and screw on the band. It should be tight and firm, but not as firm as if you were using the full force of your hands to screw it. I call it finger-strength.
4. Load the jars into the canner (with the wire rack already in the water). You also have the option of loading the jars into the wire rack first and then using the rack handles to lower it into the hot water. If you need more water to keep the water level a couple of inches above the jars, you can add hot water.
5. Turn up the heat, cover the canner with its lid, and bring the water to a vigorous boil for the amount of time called for in the recipe. It's okay to lower the heat if the boiling is excessive, but you want to keep the water at a vigorous boil. The processing time starts when your water is boiling vigorously (not when you place the jars in the hot water).

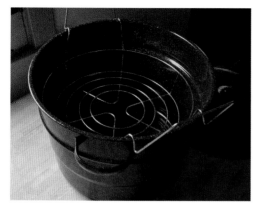

Step 1. Fill your canner with warm water, adjusting so you'll end up with a couple of inches over the tops of the jars.

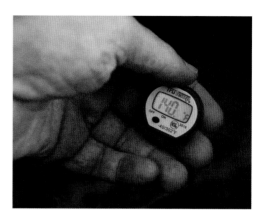

Bring your water to around 140°F (60°C).

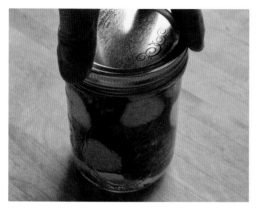

Step 2 and 3. Fill jars as per the recipe. Place the lid on each jar and screw on the band.

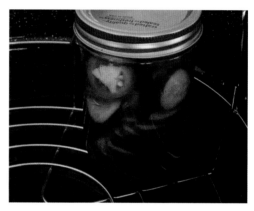

Step 4. Load the filled jars into the canner. If you need more water, you can add hot water.

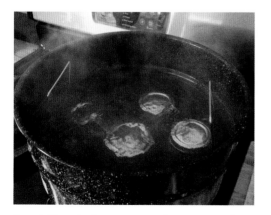

Step 5. Turn the heat up, cover the canner, and bring the water to a vigorous boil.

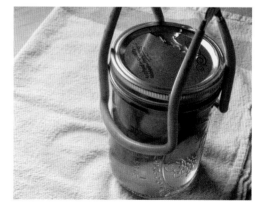

Step 7. Use a jar lifter to extract the jars one by one. Set them aside and let cool for a day or so.

6. When the jars have been processed in the boiling water for the recommended time (see "Boiling Time," turn off the heat, wait a couple of minutes, then remove the canner's lid.

7. Using the jar lifter, extract the jars one by one and set them aside. It's a good idea to place a towel underneath.

Table 7.1. Additional Processing Time Necessary Due to Altitude

Elevation above Sea Level (ft.)	Additional Processing Time (minutes)
1,001–3,000	5
3,001–6,000	10
6,001–8,000	15
8,001–10,000	20

As the jars are cooling and shrinking, a vacuum is created by the contents inside. After a while you'll hear a "pop" sound and the lid should become slightly curved down in the center. Once the jars have cooled for 12 hours, you can remove the screw band and verify that they are sealed properly by inspecting them visually. You can also gently press the middle of the lid with your finger. If the lid springs back up when you release your finger, it is an improper seal.

If the jar is improperly sealed, place it in the fridge and consume it within the next few days.

Don't forget to label the jars with the recipe and date.

Boiling Time

For the pickled wild edible recipes in this book, I use a boiling time of 15 minutes if using ½ pint (240 ml) or pint (480 ml) jars and 25 minutes if using quart (1 L) jars.

Water boils at different temperatures based on altitude. To ensure food safety and proper pasteurization, you may need to increase the boiling time asked for in the recipe based on your location. See table 7.1 for a schedule.

PICKLED RADISH PODS

This basic recipe and procedure can be applied to a large number of wild edibles, such as cattail shoots, wild onions, purslane, black mustard stems, and so on.

For canned radish pods, I usually add 1 crushed garlic clove, 1 dried chili pod, and ½ teaspoon (1.5 g) of Italian or French herb mix in each jar. Ginger also works well with pickled ingredients such as yucca (*Hesperoyucca whipplei*) shoots or mustard stems. Feel free to experiment with this very basic pickling solution, but keep the ratio of vinegar to water. You can increase or decrease the amount of sugar and salt.

Ingredients for around six ½-pint jars (1.4 L)

2 cups (480 ml) apple cider vinegar

1½ cups (360 ml) water
(white wine is also an option)

2 tablespoons (30 ml) maple syrup,
honey, or sugar

1½ teaspoons (7.5 g) sea salt

1 pound (455 g) wild radish pods

Spices and aromatic herbs of your choice
(optional)

Procedure

1. Mix the vinegar, water, maple syrup, and salt in a nonreactive bowl. Stir to dissolve the syrup and salt.
2. Loosely fill your (clean) jars with the radish pods and any spices and aromatic herbs you want to use.
3. Add the pickling vinegar solution to the jars, making sure to leave at least ½ inch (1.3 cm) headspace.
4. Preserve using the standard procedure for water bath canning (see "Water Bath Canning," page 236). I boil my jars for 15 minutes because I am at sea level, but you may need to increase your processing time based on altitude.

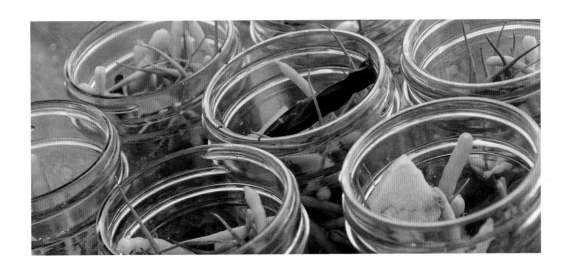

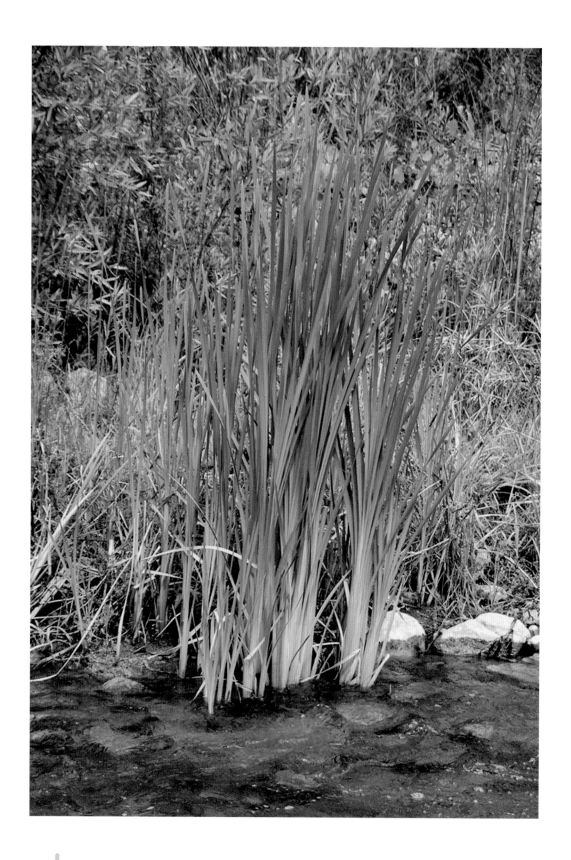

Cattail

Cattail loves wetland habitats, and it grows along the edges of lakes; in streams, marshes, and swamps; or in very wet soil. It is usually 5 to 8 feet (1.5 to 2.4 m) tall once mature. Cattail is easily recognizable with its stiff, flat leaf blades. In the center is an erect rounded stem that reaches up to 6 or 7 feet (1.8 to 2.1 m) in height. At the end of the stem, the flower head forms a cylinder that's densely packed with tiny male flowers in the top cluster and tiny female flowers in the bottom cluster. When the male cluster is loaded with pollen it looks bright yellow. The pollen, which can be used as a flour substitute, is extremely easy to forage in large quantities.

Picked at the right time of the year, every part of the plant is edible. It has countless other uses, too. The long flat leaves can be made into hats, roofing, sandals, and woven baskets. The dried leaves can be twisted to make dolls and various children's toys. I use the fibers to make cordage, as well. The seed hairs are fantastic tinder for starting fires. The crushed roots can be applied to burns, bruises, or cuts to promote healing and soothe pain.

For the recipes here, we are mostly interested in the tender stems. They look very much like leeks, and you can cook them as such. They're quite delicious when sautéed, but more often than not I just slice them and eat them raw in salads. Their flavor is similar to cucumber, but with a nutty accent.

To harvest them, I usually pull back the two main outer leaves, then grab the other inner leaves and pull gently. It is best to do this when the plant is growing in water. Depending on the season, location, and age of the plant, the first 4 to 10 inches (10 to 25 cm) are tender and edible.

It's best to forage cattail shoots in early spring, and the pollen in May or June. In Southern California we sometimes have both a fall and spring season.

However, you should know that cattails help with the remediation of polluted sites. Don't pick cattails where there is lot of human activity, horse riding, and the like, as there might be harmful chemicals, bacteria, or even parasites in the water that could compromise the plant's edibility.

PICKLED CATTAIL SHOOTS

This is a very basic recipe, but feel free to experiment with your favorite spices.

Ingredients for four
1-pint jars (1.9 L)

Around 20 medium cattail shoots

2 cups (480 ml) water or white wine

3 cups (720 ml) apple cider vinegar
   (5 percent acidity)

In each jar

2 small chili pods (optional,
   but I like a little spicy kick)

2 teaspoons (10 ml) maple syrup,
   honey, or sugar

½ teaspoon (2.5 g) sea salt

1½ teaspoons (4.5 g) pickling spices

1 sprig of sweet white clover or fresh dill

Procedure

1. Clean your cattail shoots in cold water and keep the most tender parts, usually the first 5 (12.5 cm) inches or so. Remove the outer layers if necessary. Cut the shoots to a length so they will fit in the jars (around 4¼ inches, or 11 cm).

2. Clean the jars thoroughly, then place the shoots and other ingredients in them.

3. Mix the water and vinegar to make the pickling solution and distribute it evenly in each jar, making sure to leave at least ½ inch (1.3 cm) headspace.

4. Preserve using the standard procedure for water bath canning (see "Water Bath Canning," page 236). I boil my jars for 15 minutes because I am at sea level, but you may need to increase your processing time based on altitude.

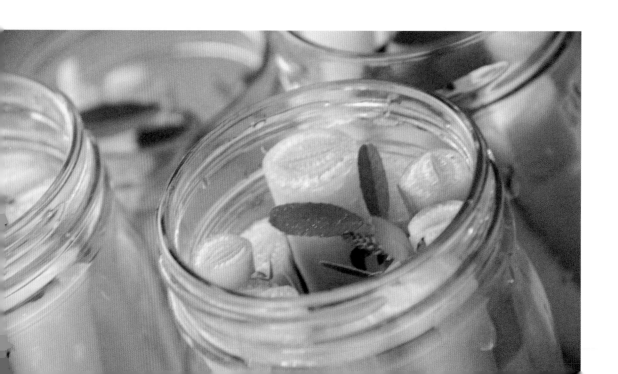

PICKLED YUCCA FLOWERS

Not all yucca flowers can be used for this recipe. I tried making it with my local chaparral yucca, but the flowers were too tender. You need thick yucca flowers similar to the ones found on datil yucca (*Yucca baccata*). The pickled flowers are delicious but also very pretty and perfect as a decorative addition to a dish.

The same recipe can be used with unopened yucca flower buds, but you'll need to double the amount, as the buds are usually half the size of the flowers.

This recipe is adapted from my first book, *The New Wildcrafted Cuisine*, in which you'll also find canning recipes for pickled yucca shoots and fruits.

Ingredients for four
1-pint jars (1.9 L)

3½ cups (840 ml) apple cider vinegar
   or white wine vinegar
2 cups (480 ml) water or white wine

In each jar

Around 30 yucca flowers
3 teaspoons (6 g) grated ginger
2½ tablespoons (37 ml) maple syrup,
   honey, or sugar
1½ teaspoons (7.5 g) salt

Procedure

1. Combine the vinegar and water and distribute evenly between the (clean) jars, making sure to leave at least ½ inch (1.3 cm) headspace.
2. Carefully detach the flowers from the stems and clean them briefly in cold water. Pat gently with a clean towel and place them into the jars. Add the ginger, maple syrup, and salt into the jars (note that the ingredients list contains the amount per jar).
3. Preserve using the standard procedure for water bath canning (see "Water Bath Canning," page 236). I boil my jars for 15 minutes because I am at sea level, but you may need to increase your processing time based on altitude.

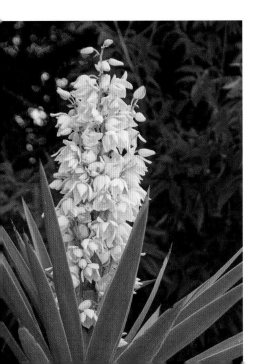
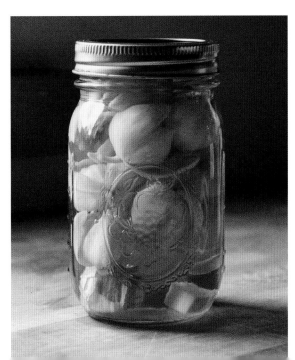

PICKLED UNRIPE WALNUTS

I think this is my favorite pickled wild ingredient. The flavor reminds me of a cross between Worcestershire sauce and A.1. steak sauce. So far, I have not found one person who doesn't like them. The process is somewhat lengthy, but it's so worth it!

The recipe is based on a traditional British recipe. I've prepared it with various types of unripe black walnuts found on the West Coast, as well as with unripe Persian walnuts, which grow "feral" around Los Angeles but are the same ones you buy at the store. This recipe is also in my first book, *The New Wildcrafted Cuisine*, along with a similar recipe for pickled acorns.

Some people on the East Coast who tried making this recipe told me that their native walnuts ended up too mushy. If that's the case, you might try using a blender to make a sort of savory walnut paste instead of using the whole walnuts as a condiment. Some black walnuts trees are becoming rare around Los Angeles due to urban expansion and habitat destruction. As a wildcrafter, I always make a point of growing and planting several trees, including black walnut, each year.

Pickled black walnuts get much better with age. The minimum amount of time you should wait before consuming is a month, but I think they're much better after at least 6 months or even more. I'm currently enjoying a batch that is 2 years old.

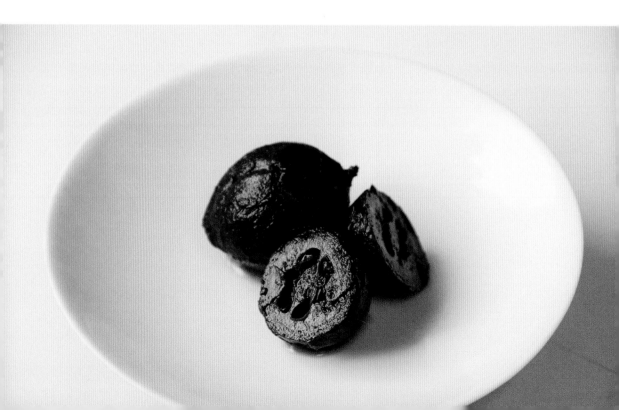

Materials

Boiling water bath canner

Glass preserving jars, lids, and bands

2- to 3-gallon bucket

Jar lifter

Home canning funnel

Thermometer

Bucket for brining

Plate

Rock to use as weight

Small wooden board with a nail,
 to puncture the nuts

Ingredients for about six 1-pint jars (2.9 L)

Around 2⅔ pounds (1.2 kg) unripe walnuts,
 see step #1

2 cups (480 g) salt, divided

20 cups (4.8 L) water, divided

1 cup (240 ml) white wine

2 cups (480 ml) red wine vinegar

½ cup (120 ml) balsamic vinegar

1 cup (220 g) brown sugar

In each jar

1½ teaspoons (4.5 g) garlic powder

1 teaspoon (2 g) grated ginger

1 teaspoon (3 g) Italian herbs blend
 or herbes de Provence blend

½ teaspoon (2 g) peppercorns

½ California bay leaf or 1 regular bay leaf

4 whole cloves

Dried chilies (optional)

Procedure

1. Forage the walnuts while the shell is still soft inside (late spring). If the shell is already hard, it's too late. Before you collect a bunch of nuts, use a knife to test a few, evaluating whether they're good for pickling. The knife should slice through the shell easily (like a potato) and you should see the unripe walnut inside. Wear gloves! The walnut juice can stain your skin.

2. You'll need to poke holes in each unripe walnut so the brine and pickling solution can permeate the inside of the nut. It also allows the walnuts to release their juice. I usually use a little wooden board with a nail to puncture the nuts. I place a walnut between my fingers and make around 6 to 8 holes in each. I can process around 10 to 12 walnuts a minute this way. Again, wear gloves, as it is a messy business and you can end up with stained fingers. Yes, you'll probably poke your fingers from time to time in the beginning, but with experience you'll get better.

3. Combine 1 cup (240 g) of the salt and 10 cups (2.4 L) of the water to form a brine. Boil the brine so the water is well saturated with the salt, then cool it down. Place the walnuts in a 2- to 3-gallon (7.5 to 11.3 L) bucket and pour enough brine to cover them. Make sure the walnuts are under the surface of the brine. I use a plate with a boiled (pasteurized) rock on top to keep them submerged. Once the walnuts are saturated with salt, they will not float, but this could take days.

4. Leave the walnuts in the brine for around 10 days. Shake or stir the contents once a day. After a couple of days, the surface of the brine will look like some sort of toxic waste. Don't worry, you're doing fine. Nothing bad is happening under the surface scum.

5. Drain the brine, rinse the walnuts very briefly, and replace the old brine with a new one using the same salt to water ratio.

6. Wait 10 more days, shaking or stirring once a day.

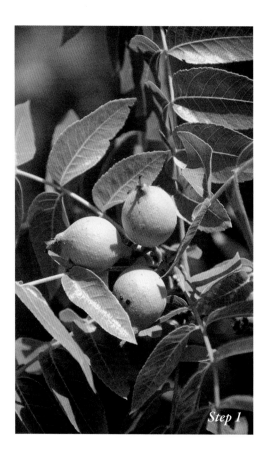

Step 1

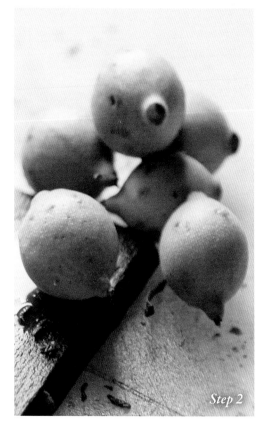

Step 2

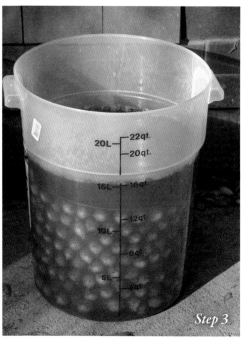

Step 3

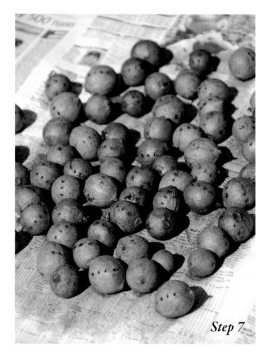

Step 7

246 Wildcrafted Vinegars

7. Remove the walnuts from the brine. Rinse them briefly with regular tap water and place them in the sun. In Southern California where the sun is strong, they can turn jet black by the end of the day. In another region, where the sun isn't as strong, this might take a couple of days. Once they're jet black, they are ready for pickling.

8. Make the pickling solution by combining the wine, vinegars, and brown sugar in a small pot. Bring the solution to a boil, then remove from heat.

9. Gather the jars you will use. There is no need to sterilize the jars since you will be placing them in a boiling-water bath for more than 10 minutes. Just clean them with soap and water.

10. Place the spices into each jar.

11. Fill the jars with your black walnuts. Pour the hot pickling solution inside the jar, leaving a ½ inch (1.3 cm) headspace, and tighten the lids to "finger strength."

12. Preheat the water in the water bath canner to 180°F (82°C). You'll want enough water to cover the jars by at least 1 inch (2.5 cm). Use the jar lifter to place the jars in the canner.

13. Place the lid on the water bath canner and bring water to a rolling boil.

14. Process the pint jars for 25 minutes in the boiling water (time starts when the boiling begins). Increase the processing time based on your altitude if necessary (see table 7.1 page 238). When complete, shut off heat and remove the canner's lid. Allow the jars to rest in the canner for 5 minutes.

15. Remove the jars from the water with the jar lifter and set on a towel. Verify that you have achieved a proper vacuum inside; the lids should make a popping sound as the jars cool. Let the jars cool completely (12 hours). Check the seal the next day by pressing on the center of the lids; they should not bounce back.

16. Store in a cool, dark place. The walnuts should keep for a couple of years in the right storage conditions.

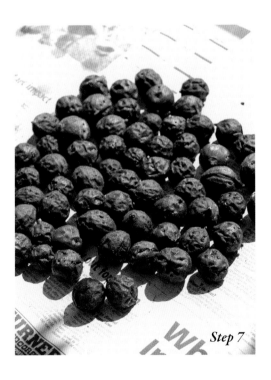

Step 7

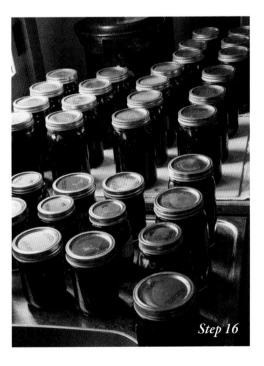

Step 16

Vinegar in Soups

It may sound a bit strange and unusual for some, but vinegar is a common ingredient in some soup recipes, and there is a good reason for it. If you think about it, vinegar is really a flavor-enhancer (umami). That's why it is so often used in cooking, sauces, and salad dressings. The same is true with soups.

Some good examples are the classic Chinese sweet, hot, and sour soups and sauces, but you'll find vinegar used in recipes from numerous other countries and cultures, as well.

So, a big YES to vinegars in soups! To be honest, this was kind of a new concept for me before working on this book, but these days I often use vinegar in my wild food soups.

In this book, I want to share a very, very basic vinegar soup stock recipe that anyone can make. With it, I'm able to make a comforting soup in minutes using the plants from any hike. The secret code for this soup stock is 1.1.1.

The 1.1.1. Soups

The simple soup stock is composed of:

> 1 cup (240 ml) soup stock or water (boiling hot)
> 1 tablespoon (15 ml) soy sauce
> 1 tablespoon (15 ml) vinegar (spicy ones are the best!)

That's it. Now of course, it's much better with a good soup stock (plant-based or not), but even water works. If you only have water, maybe add a teaspoon of blended herbs and fresh onion/garlic in the bowl, but water alone will still be okay.

You have tons of creative possibilities. The vinegar can be homemade and spicy (like Tabasco), for example, but what you put in the bowl is also endlessly creative. Go on a hike, pick some of your favorite wild edibles, and use them alongside regular savory ingredients such as garlic, onion, chili peppers, and so on. For the soup in the photo I used fermented burdock roots, pickled radish pods, nettles pasta, minced black mustard leaves, sliced red onion, garlic, and ½ teaspoon (1.5 g) of Italian herbs. I like to cut the wild greens in small strips (chiffonade) so that even tough leaves become edible.

So seriously, try it. . . . I think you'll love it. It's perfect for foragers who can collect various savory plants to make something quick and delicious, but it obviously works with store-bought ingredients, too. If you're a fermenter, you can add some of your favorite savory ferments like I did with

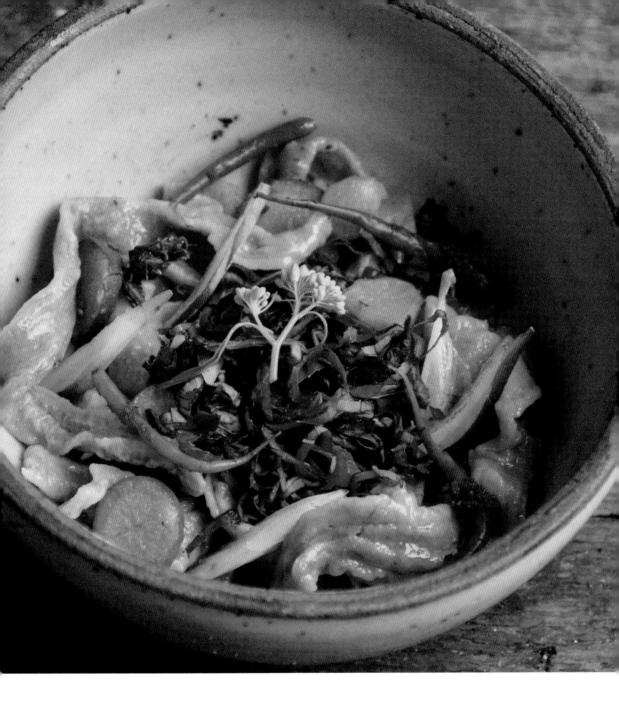

the fermented burdock roots. Oh . . . and seaweed! Seaweed with sliced red onions and tofu . . . so good!

If it's too salty for you, reduce the amount of soy sauce. And try a good spicy vinegar or a vinegar-based hot sauce like Tabasco. Such a nice balance. If you use Tabasco, make it half regular cider vinegar and half Tabasco, otherwise it might be too spicy. The following 2 recipes are examples to show the versatility.

MIXED SEASONAL WILD GREENS AND MUSHROOMS SOUP

With this kind of soup (1.1.1., page 248), you can easily take advantage of what's in season in your environment. In Southern California I've always found wild greens I could use at any time of the year, such as watercress, chickweed, wild mustard leaves, miner's lettuce, and so on. Even during the winter, I was able to use young mustard or wild radish sprouts.

In this recipe I'm using commercial baby bella mushrooms. If you use foraged mushrooms, make sure to cook them first. Some wild mushrooms, such as morels, can be toxic if they are eaten raw or not fully cooked.

Ingredients for 1 large bowl (240 ml)

1½ cups (360 ml) soup stock or water
¼ onion, sliced
2 tablespoons (7 g) chopped wild greens
1½ tablespoons (23 ml) soy sauce
1½ tablespoons (23 ml) homemade vinegar
of your choice or apple cider vinegar
1 baby bella mushroom, sliced
1 dry chili pepper
½ garlic clove, minced

Procedure

Place a pot containing the soup stock over high heat and bring to a boil.

Meanwhile, place all the remaining ingredients into a bowl. If you use wild mushrooms, make sure to cook them first.

Pour the boiling stock over the ingredients and wait 5 or 6 minutes before serving. If you want to keep the soup very warm, you can place a plate on top of the bowl.

This kind of soup is quick and easy to make, which was perfect for my classes. We were able to do a wild food walk, collect wild greens, and make a soup on the spot.

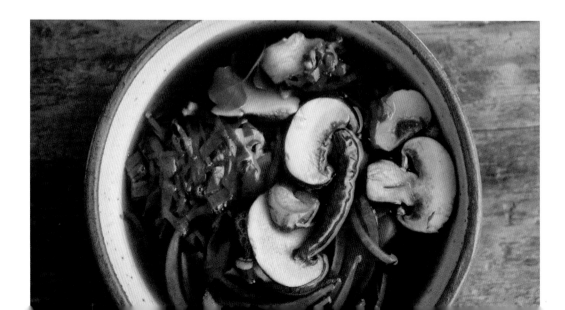

WILD RADISH ROOTS SOUP

This is another example of the versatility of the 1.1.1 soup (page 248). You're not stuck using just common wild greens and mushrooms. There are all kinds of savory or nutritious ingredients that can be added, such as roots, seeds and grains, edible flowers, and even insects. I used to have a small mealworm "farm" in my apartment and would sometimes add dehydrated mealworms to my soups as a source of protein and nutty flavor.

The Brassica family has a lot of edible roots. Personally, I've used wild radish, black mustard, and Mediterranean mustard roots to make this kind of soup. Realize that timing is important, as a lot of the wild Brassica roots become tough and fibrous over time. Feel free to create other soups around this basic recipe by adding ingredients from your own terroir.

Ingredients for 1 large bowl (240 ml)

1½ cups (360 ml) soup stock or water

¼ onion, sliced

2 to 3 wild radish pods

3 to 4 small and tender wild radish
   or mustard roots

1½ tablespoons (23 ml) soy sauce

1½ tablespoons (23 ml) homemade vinegar
   of your choice or apple cider vinegar

½ jalapeño, sliced

½ garlic clove, minced

1 teaspoon (4 g) wild oat grains (I cook them
   well in advance and freeze them)

1 teaspoon (1.9 g) sliced black mustard stems

Procedure

Place a pot containing the soup stock over high heat and bring to a boil. Meanwhile, place all the remaining ingredients into a bowl.

Pour the boiling water over the ingredients and wait 5 or 6 minutes before serving. If you want to keep the soup very warm, you can place a plate on top of the bowl.

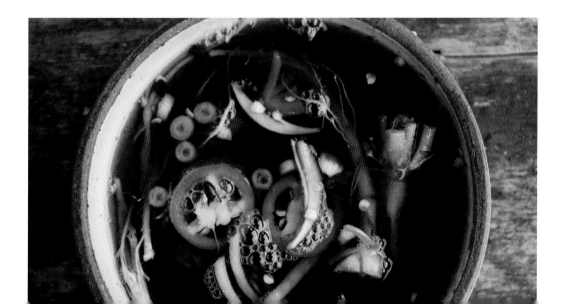

RAW VINEGAR SOUP: GAZPACHO

Gazpacho is a traditional raw, cold soup originating from the Iberian Peninsula and still commonly eaten in Portugal and Spain during the hot summer months. Even in Belgium, my mom used to have her own version using vegetables from our garden.

Raw vinegar soup is quite nutritious and refreshing. A good homemade vinegar brings it to a new level. This kind of soup is perfect for springtime wild edibles such as miner's lettuce, chervil, wild mustard sprouts, or chickweed. You can play with this basic recipe by using or adding other ingredients such as celery, avocados, grapes, Tabasco, croutons, and so on.

Ingredients for 2 to 3 servings

3 large tomatoes (see Note)
0.5 ounce (14 g) chopped red onion
0.5 ounce (14 g) chopped bell pepper
    (yellow or orange)
¼ cup (14 g) minced wild greens
    or store-bought greens
    (parsley or cilantro)
1 Roma tomato, chopped
1 garlic clove, minced
½ jalapeño, chopped
1 tablespoon (9 g) sliced wild
    or store-bought green onion
1 cucumber, chopped
2 tablespoons (30 ml) Apple Scraps Vinegar
    or unpasteurized apple cider vinegar
1 teaspoon (5 ml) Tabasco-style spicy vinegar
    or Tabasco hot sauce (optional)
2 teaspoons (10 ml) A.1. steak sauce
    or Worcestershire sauce
Salt and pepper to taste

Procedure

Clean, chop, and place the 3 large tomatoes in a food processor until smooth. You should end up with around 2 cups (480 ml) of liquid.

In a large bowl, toss together the onion, bell pepper, wild greens, Roma tomato, garlic, jalapeño, green onion, and cucumber. Add the pureed tomatoes, vinegar, Tabasco and A.1. steak sauce.

Gently stir the contents and place in the refrigerator for an hour or so before serving. Taste and add salt or pepper if necessary

My favorite vinegars for this soup are Smoked Mushroom–Infused Vinegar, homemade apple cider vinegar, or red wine vinegar.

Note: *Many traditional recipes use strained tomato juice instead of pureed tomatoes. Pureed tomatoes are strictly my own personal preference and make the soup chunkier.*

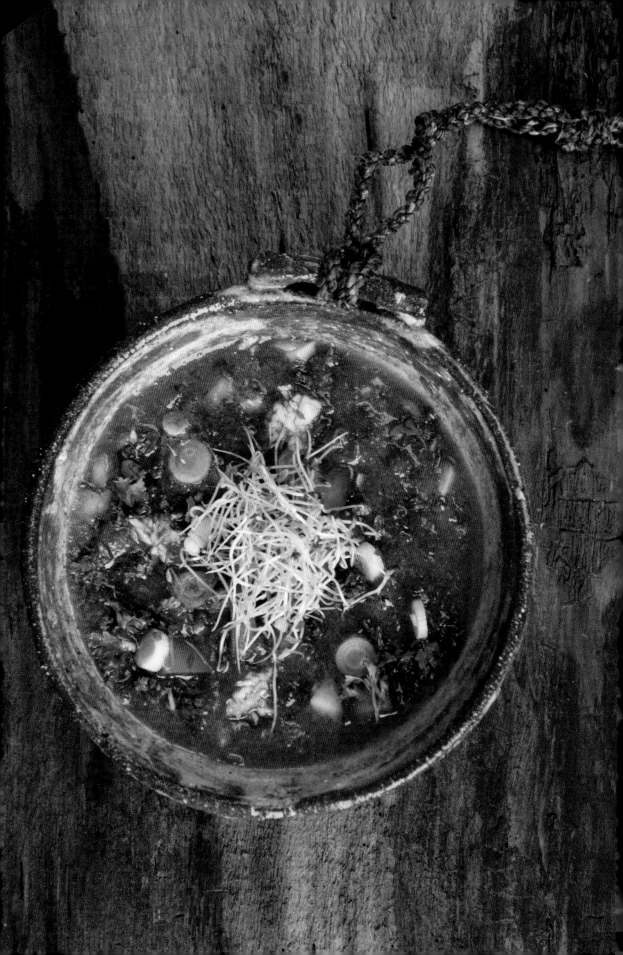

Vinegar Drinks

Nowadays, most people don't associate vinegar with tasty drinks. This is kind of interesting because in most supermarkets you'll find all sorts of flavored kombucha drinks, which are similarly sour and tangy.

But if you go back in history, vinegar-based drinks were once very common. In ancient Greece, oxycrate was one of the main beverages for the common people. It was a simple mixture of water, honey, and vinegar—quite refreshing and medicinal, as well. Vinegar was touted by Hippocrates, the "Father of Medicine," as a treatment for all kinds of ailments such as wounds, infections, coughs, and so on.

But the Greeks were not alone. The Romans had a similar drink, called posca. Posca was again the main drink of the common people, but also the standard drink for the Roman army. Flavors aside, I think the use of vinegar-based drinks in antiquity made a lot of sense, as some sources of water could be iffy. The acetic acid in vinegar could probably help reduce the amount of common germs such as *E. coli* or salmonella. But that's my own speculation. I have never seen a scientific study on that subject for vinegar-based drinks.

Although the exact recipe for posca was unwritten, based on historical bits and pieces culinary historians think it went something like this:

INGREDIENTS FOR A 1-QUART JAR (1 L)

2¾ cups (660 ml) water
1 cup (240 ml) red wine vinegar
⅓ cup (80 ml) honey
2 teaspoons (3.5 g) coriander seeds

PROCEDURE

Mix all the ingredients and bring the contents to a boil.
Remove from heat, let it cool down, and strain. It's now ready to
    drink. Stored in the fridge, this beverage will keep for weeks.

Vinegar-based drinks seem to have slowly gone out of fashion during the Middle Ages, although *sekanjabin*—a sweet Persian beverage made of vinegar, sugar or honey, water, limes, cucumber, mint, and water—was still popular at the time.

In the 17th century there was a slight renaissance. The English shrub, a sort of upcycled vinegar drink, arose and was eventually adopted in colonial America. Shrubs originated as a byproduct of food preservation.

Berries and fruits collected during summer and fall would be preserved in jars filled with vinegar. Once the berries were eaten, the flavored vinegar that remained would be mixed with maple syrup, honey, or sugar, then reduced to make a syrup. The syrup would then be mixed into either water or carbonated water and served as a tasty, refreshing drink. During the same period, you would also find switchel, *honeygar*, and oxymel.

If you research each of these beverages, you'll notice the common ingredients of vinegar, a sugary base, and water. You'll notice, too, that the flavoring will vary immensely through the uses of savory herbs, spices, berries, and fruits.

To make the differentiation simpler, shrubs tend to be made from fruits and berries and possibly spices and herbs. Switchel is a honey and vinegar drink that often has ginger as a main flavoring base. Honeygar is boiled water combined with honey and vinegar. Oxymel (also a blend of honey and vinegar) is much more herbal. Some oxymel recipes, created by herbalists, have medicinal purposes.

This is a very quick and incomplete history. I'll be honest, I don't care too much about the various labels and what my drinks should be called. Working with my local

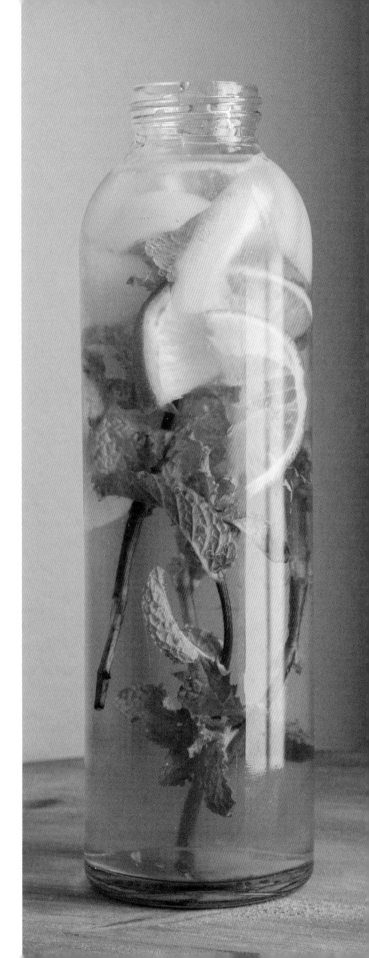

environment, I often mix fruits, spices, and herbs in my vinegar drinks in such a way that you would have a hard time placing a specific label on them. I just call them vinegar drinks or tonics.

In modern times, mostly among the health-conscious public, we've seen a slight revival of vinegar drinks for their possible medicinal properties, but also for their taste. Maybe one day kombucha will fall out of favor and be replaced by vinegar tonics. Who knows!

If you make your own raw (wild) vinegars at home, you can create unique and incredibly tasty probiotic drinks that are a representation of your terroir. For example, last week I made a simple vinegar drink with Elderberry Wine Vinegar, manzanita powder (a local berry that tastes like sweet apples), maple syrup, water, and a touch of lime juice. It was delicious, but would be impossible to purchase in a supermarket.

The pages that follow feature a couple of simple recipes you can try with store-bought ingredients to get you started, and from there you can experiment with wilder versions.

I typically use 1 of 4 methods to make my vinegar drinks:

1. Fresh fruits and berries, which usually requires blending and straining
2. Homemade fruit or berry juice, with or without herbal additions
3. Savory infused vinegars
4. Cold infusions of fresh herbal ingredients

And of course, you can mix the various methods. For example, mix an infused vinegar with fresh berries or juice. There are no rules!

BASIC APPLE CIDER TONIC

This tonic is easy to make and quite delicious. There is a lot of room for creativity by expanding on this basic recipe with spices, tasty fruit syrups, and even fresh juice.

Ingredients for a 1-pint jar (480 ml)

1¾ cups (420 ml) water

1 tablespoon (15 ml) raw apple cider vinegar

1 tablespoon (15 ml) fresh lime juice

1 tablespoon (15 ml) maple syrup,
    honey, or sugar

1 teaspoon (2 g) freshly grated ginger

3 to 4 bruised sprigs organic mint (optional)

Procedure

Place all the ingredients in a jar and shake for a few seconds. Store in the refrigerator and serve cold. It should keep for several days.

JUICE-BASED VINEGAR TONICS

Simplicity itself, and yet so many possibilities. If you make the juice from wildcrafted ingredients, use these recipes as guidelines. You will proceed using your taste buds due to the wide variation of sweetness in wild berries and fruits. When I make a new recipe, I usually mix all of my ingredients, then slowly add maple syrup or honey and taste as I go along.

You can also use already-made organic juices or purchase fruits and berries from the store or farmers market, and then make your own juice.

Basic Grape Vinegar Tonic

Ingredients for a 1-quart jar (1 L)

2½ cups (600 ml) water

1 cup (240 ml) homemade grape juice
    or store-bought organic grape juice
    (no sugar added)

2 tablespoons (30 ml) apple cider vinegar

2 tablespoons (30 ml) maple syrup, honey,
    or organic sugar

Procedure

Place all the ingredients in a quart (1 L) jar and shake or stir the contents until the syrup is dissolved. Store in the fridge, where it should keep for at least a week. Serve with ice. Note that some wild grapes can be very sour and you many need to add more sugar to offset.

Elderberry Vinegar Tonic

Ingredients for a 1-quart jar (1 L)

2 cups (480 ml) water

1 cup (240 ml) elderberry or blackberry juice
(foraged or store-bought), see Note

3 tablespoons (45 ml) red wine vinegar or
Elderberry Wine Vinegar

2 tablespoons (30 ml) maple syrup, honey,
or organic sugar

½ teaspoon (1 g) grated ginger

Procedure

Place all the ingredients in a quart jar and shake or stir the contents until the syrup is dissolved. Store in the fridge, where it should keep for at least a week. Serve with ice.

> *Note: Elderberry juice needs to be boiled before consumption. I usually boil the juice for 30 minutes and make a concentrate, then add water later to reconstitute. You can find recipes for elderberry juice or syrup online. Raw elderberry juice can make you sick.*

Local Mountains Vinegar Tonic

Some recipes look simple and yet incorporate a large number of savory herbs, berries, and plants. For example, it takes close to 12 ingredients to create the Mountains Vinegar, which I use in this recipe.

Ingredients for a 1-quart jar (1 L)

2½ cups (600 ml) water

3 tablespoons (45 ml) Mountains Vinegar

2 tablespoons (30 ml) pinyon pine cone syrup
(see *The Wildcrafting Brewer*) or maple syrup

1 tablespoon (15 ml) fresh lime juice

1 sprig of white fir in each glass for garnish
(cut the tip of the needles to increase
flavor extraction)

Procedure

Place all the ingredients except the white fir sprigs in a quart jar and shake or stir the contents until the syrup is dissolved. Store in the fridge, where it should keep for at least a week. Serve with ice and a white fir sprig.

FRESH BERRIES VINEGAR DRINK

This recipe will work with all kinds of foraged berries—blackberries, blue-berries, wild currants, cranberries, and so on. But realize that you'll need to adjust the sweetness based on the berries you are using. For example, if you are using cranberries, you'll need to add more maple syrup or honey to the recipe in order to balance the sourness of the berries.

You can use store-bought ingredients, but if you are a wildcrafter, you'll realize that many store-bought berries are truly lacking in taste compared to their wild counterparts. I purchased some blue-berries yesterday and they were completely tasteless. You may need to increase the number of berries or even add some juice to make up for the lack of flavor.

A typical ingredients list would look like this (for 1 quart, or 1 L):

2¾ cups (660 ml) water
½ to ¾ cup (120 to 180 ml by volume) wild
    or commercial berries
2 to 3 tablespoons (30 to 45 ml) apple cider
    vinegar or vinegar of your choice
2 tablespoons (30 ml) maple syrup, honey,
    or sugar, more (or less) as needed

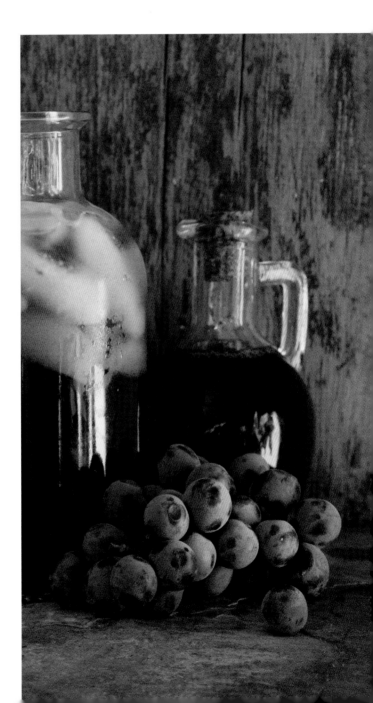

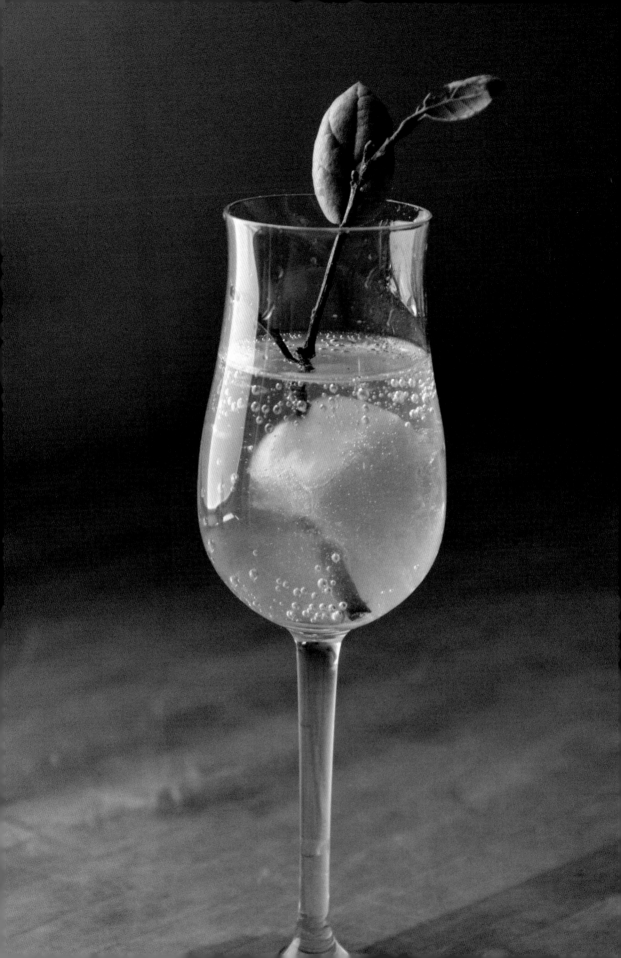

MOUNTAIN OXYMEL,
AKA "MOUNTAIN CHAMPAGNE"

The infused vinegar that I use for this recipe is composed mostly of plants, so I think I'm correct in calling this an oxymel. But I usually refer to it as my "mountain champagne." It's my favorite wild vinegar drink so far. It tastes like the local mountains—pine, lemon, tangerine, sagebrush, bittersweet. It's superbly complex in terms of flavors.

Recipes for infused vinegars can be found in chapter 3, and for this drink any pine-, fir-, or spruce-infused vinegar would work nicely. The concept is very straightforward: Make a syrup with 50 percent sugar, maple syrup, or honey and 50 percent of your favorite infused vinegar, then add carbonated water when you want to enjoy.

Ingredients for a 1-pint jar (480 ml) of syrup

1 cup (240 ml) infused vinegar
  of your choice
1 cup (240 ml) honey, maple syrup,
  or organic cane sugar
Carbonated water to serve

Procedure

Strain your infused vinegar (if it has not yet been strained), pour it in a medium saucepan, and add the honey.

Bring the liquid to a boil, then simmer for a minute or so. If you used sugar, make sure it is fully dissolved. Stir if necessary.

Strain the liquid, let it cool, then pour the contents into a clean pint jar (½ L) or bottle. Screw the lid on tightly or cork the bottle. Store in the refrigerator or in a cool, dark place. This is a very acidic syrup that will keep well for months.

When ready to use, place some ice cubes in a glass and pour enough vinegar syrup to fill between 15 to 25 percent of the volume. Fill the rest of the glass with carbonated water and voila! Your "champagne" is ready.

Note: There are huge numbers of creative drinks you can make with this technique. You could even make a tasty syrup by simmering some regular apple cider vinegar and sugar with the addition of fruits, berries, and spices.

COLD INFUSION FOREST
VINEGAR TONIC

I used to make this type of drink for some of the restaurants I worked with. It is basically a fresh herbal infusion that is placed in the refrigerator overnight or for a couple of days at the most. The idea behind the cold infusion is to minimize potential bacteria growth, which can occur at regular temperatures.

The principle is quite basic: Chop or bruise some tasty wildcrafted herbs; add vinegar, lemons, and sugar or honey; then place the container in the refrigerator. The herbs will slowly release their flavors. I usually serve it at my classes or workshops in a lemonade jar with a spigot.

The true art is in creating a beautiful and delicious blend. With experience and plant knowledge, you can create incredible beverages to represent specific environments, such as your local forest or mountains. It's not unusual for me to have over 15 different ingredients that are a representation of a specific environment, a concept similar to my Mountains Vinegar.

But let's keep it simple here. While writing this book in my RV, I did a quick hike in the local forest and made this forest tonic with a few plants I collected.

Ingredients for a 1-gallon jar (4 L)

0.5 ounce (14 g) young wild oats, chopped

1 sprig horehound

4 to 5 California mugwort leaves

2 bunches (1.4 ounces, or 40 g) water mint
   or organic spearmint

¾ gallon (3 L) water

⅓ cup (80 ml) raw apple cider vinegar

⅓ cup (80 ml) maple syrup, honey, or sugar
   (you can use less or more)

1½ organic lemons, sliced
   (or limes or oranges)

Procedure

Briefly clean your oats and herbs in cold water. Bruise them gently with your fingers, which will facilitate flavor extraction, and place them in the jar. The mint can be chopped.

Add the water, vinegar, and maple syrup.

Place the lemon slices in the solution.

Close the jar and store in the fridge overnight.

Strain and serve. Sometimes, during private dinners or wild food tasting events, I keep the jar in the middle of the table for aesthetic value. In such cases, I often replace the contents with new fresh herbs.

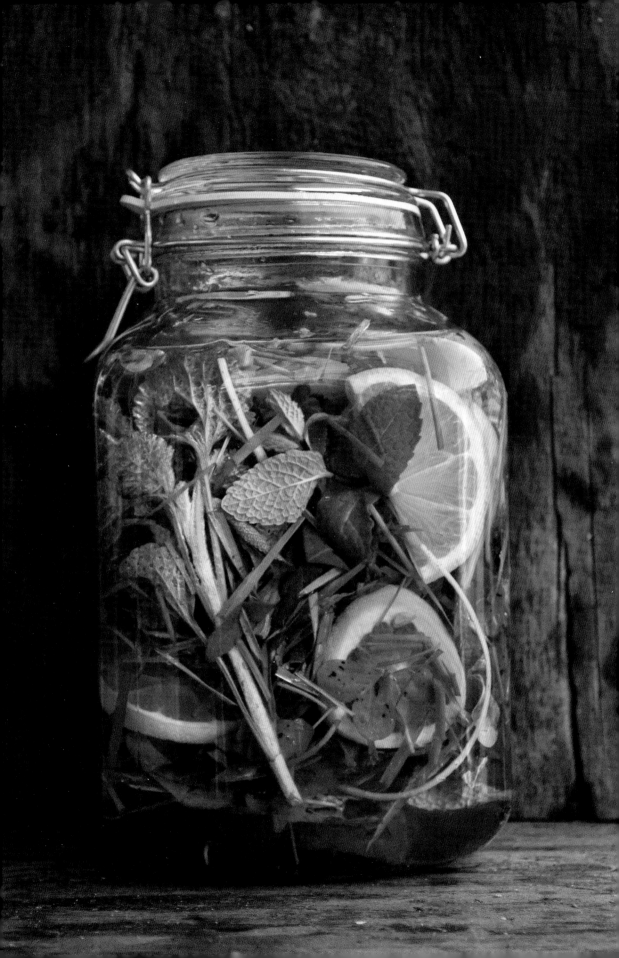

WILD GRAPES VINEGAR TONIC

I found some wild grapes in an abandoned town in the local mountains. They were extremely sweet, similar to Concord grapes, and probably planted in a garden originally. This recipe would work well with Concord grapes. If your grapes have seeds, you'll need to strain the blended contents.

Ingredients for a 1-quart jar (1 L)

2½ (600 ml) cups water

½ cup (100 g) sweet wild grapes
   or Concord grapes

2 tablespoons red wine vinegar or
   Elderberry Wine Vinegar

½ teaspoon (1 g) grated ginger (optional)

1 tablespoon (15 ml) maple syrup
   (or to taste)

Procedure

Place all the ingredients, except the maple syrup, into a blender.

Blend at medium speed and strain the contents. You can skip straining if your grapes are seedless. Taste and add maple syrup as desired.

Transfer the contents to a quart (1 L) jar, close the top, and store in the refrigerator where it will keep for at least a week.

Serve cold with some ice. This drink is very refreshing during the summer.

APPENDIX

Some of the most common edible wild plants used in this book

As a wildcrafter, you must properly identify and research any plant you intend to use. For some practical advice to get you started, see "Infusing Whole Environments" on page 116.

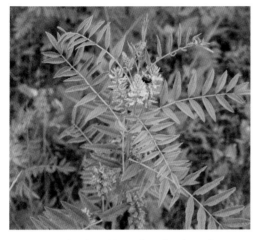

American Licorice (*Glycyrrhiza lepidota*). Roots used to infuse vinegars.

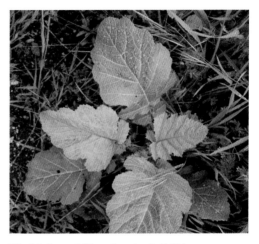

Black Mustard (*Brassica nigra*). Edible parts: roots, leaves, flowers, and seeds. Wasabi flavors.

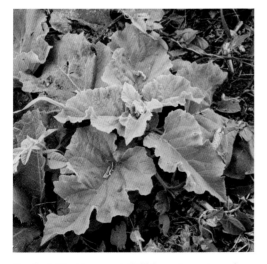

Burdock (*Arctium* spp.). Edible parts: roots and young stems.

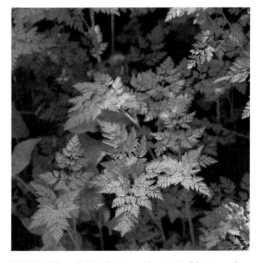

(Wild) Chervil (*Anthriscus sylvestris*). Plant used as a savory edible green.

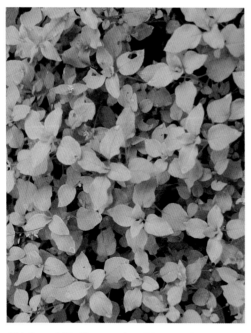

Chickweed (*Stellaria media*). Plant used as a savory edible green.

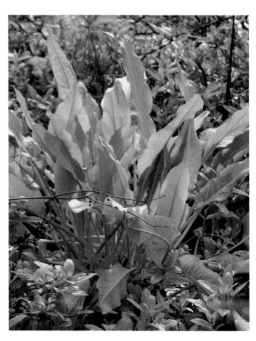

Curly Dock (*Rumex crispus*). Leaves and stems used mostly in soups or for pickled stems, in this book.

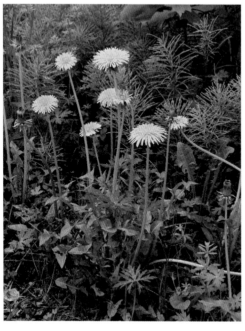

Dandelion (*Taraxacum officinale*). Leaves used in salads and soups. Bitter flavor.

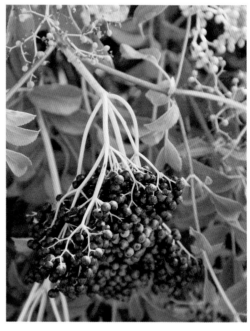

Elderberry (*Sambucus* spp.). Berries used to make wine and to infuse vinegars.

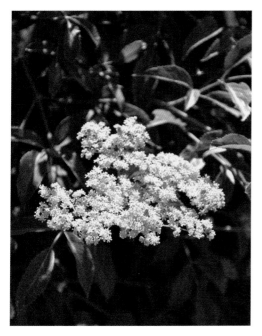

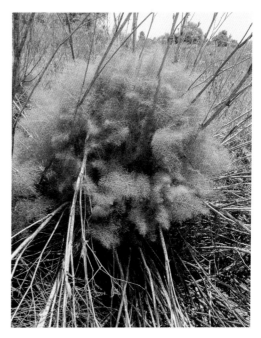

Elderflower (*Sambucus* spp.). Flowers used to flavor some alcoholic drinks or to infuse vinegars.

(Wild) Fennel (*Foeniculum vulgare*). Seeds used as a spice. Fronds and stalks used to infuse vinegars or as a savory wild green.

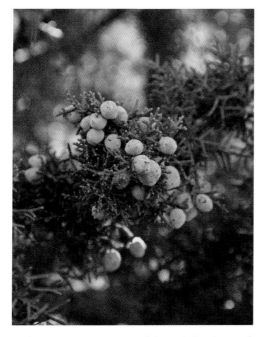

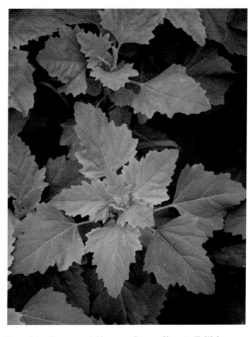

Juniper Berries (*Juniperus californica*). Berries used to infuse vinegars or as a good source of wild yeast.

Lamb's-Quarter (*Chenopodium album*). Edible parts: seeds, cooked leaves and young stems. Similar uses as spinach.

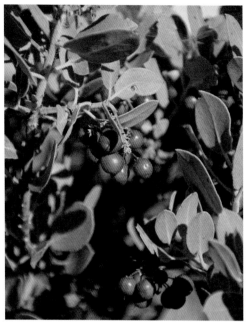

Manzanita (*Arctostaphylos manzanita*). Berries used to make fermented drinks or to infuse vinegars. Apple flavor.

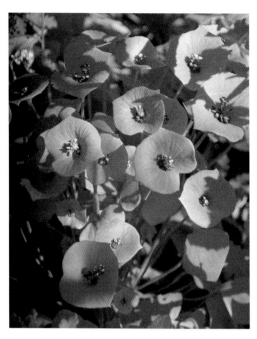

Miner's Lettuce (*Claytonia perfoliata*). Plant used as a savory edible green.

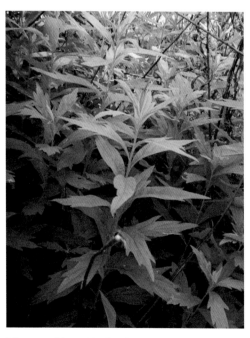

Mugwort (*Artemisia douglasiana*). Plant used as a bittering ingredient in wild beers and to infuse flavors in drinks and vinegars.

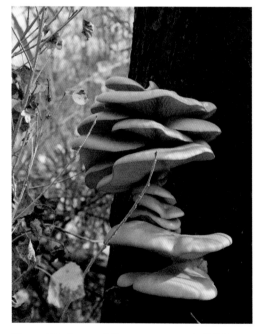

Oyster Mushroom (*Pleurotus ostreatus*). Edible mushroom sold commercially and also found in the wild.

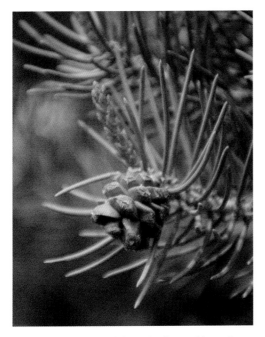

Pinyon Pine (*Pinus edulis*). Needles and branches used to infuse vinegars. Unripe pine cones are a source of wild yeast.

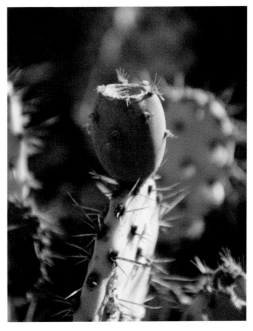

Prickly Pears (*Opuntia littoralis*). Edible fruits used for alcoholic fermentation and to make vinegars.

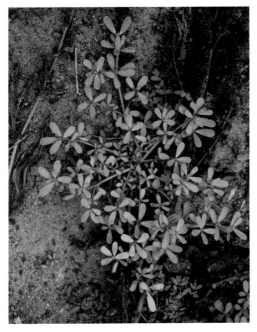

Purslane (*Portulaca oleracea*). Plant used as a savory edible green. Pickled stems are a traditional side dish in some countries.

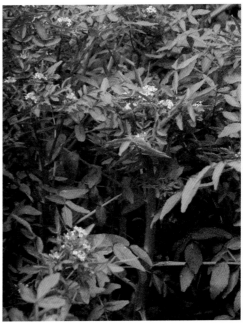

Watercress (*Nasturtium officinale*). Plant used as a savory edible green, raw or cooked.

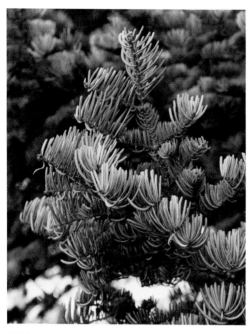

White Fir (*Abies concolor*). Needles used to infuse drinks and vinegars.

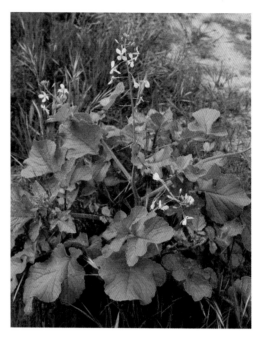

Wild Radish (*Raphanus raphanistrum*). Edible parts: roots, leaves, flowers, and tender seed pods.

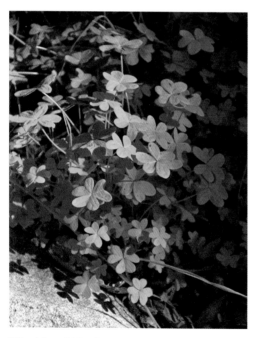

Wood Sorrel (*Oxalis* spp.). Edible parts: flowers and leaves. Very sour with lemony flavors.

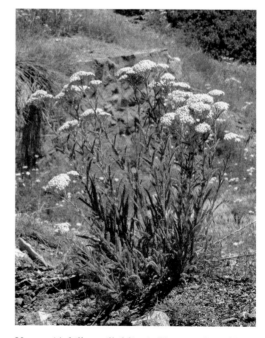

Yarrow (*Achillea millefolium*). Plant used as a bittering ingredient in wild beers and to infuse flavors in drinks and vinegars.

RESOURCES

Vinegar Making and Recipes

Vinegar Revival: Artisanal Recipes for Brightening Dishes and Drinks with Homemade Vinegars by Harry Rosenblum

Homebrewed Vinegar: How to Ferment 60 Delicious Varieties, Including Carrot-Ginger, Beet, Brown Banana, Pineapple, Corncob, Honey, and Apple Cider Vinegar by Kirsten K. Shockey

The Artisanal Vinegar Maker's Handbook: Crafting Quality Vinegars— Fermenting, Distilling, Infusing by Bettina Malle and Helge Schmickl

The Olive Oil and Vinegar Lover's Cookbook: Revised and Updated Edition by Emily Lycopolus

Asian Pickles: Sweet, Sour, Salty, Cured, and Fermented Preserves from Korea, Japan, China, India, and Beyond by Karen Solomon

Alcoholic Fermentation

Sacred and Herbal Healing Beers: The Secrets of Ancient Fermentation by Stephen Harrod Buhner

Radical Brewing: Recipes, Tales and World-Altering Meditations in a Glass by Randy Mosher

Ale, Beer, and Brewsters in England: Women's Work in a Changing World: 1300–1600 by Judith M. Bennett

Uncorking the Past: The Quest for Wine, Beer, and Other Alcoholic Beverages by Patrick E. McGovern

Make Mead Like a Viking: Traditional Techniques for Brewing Natural, Wild-Fermented, Honey-Based Wines and Beers by Jereme Zimmerman

Wild Fermentation: The Flavor, Nutrition, and Craft of Live-Culture Foods, 2nd Edition, by Sandor Ellix Katz

The Wildcrafting Brewer: Creating Unique Drinks and Boozy Concoctions from Nature's Ingredients by Pascal Baudar

Books about Plant Identification in the United States

This list includes a few books I'm familiar with, but it's very incomplete. A simple search online or on Amazon.com should help you find plant identification books you can use to learn about your local wild edible plants.

SOUTHWEST

Foraging California: Finding, Identifying, and Preparing Edible Wild Foods in California by Christopher Nyerges

The Forager's Harvest: A Guide to Identifying, Harvesting, and Preparing Edible Wild Plants by Samuel Thayer

California Foraging: 120 Wild and Flavorful Edibles from Evergreen Huckleberries to Wild Ginger by Judith Larner Lowry

Nuts and Berries of California: Tips and Recipes for Gatherers by Christopher Nyerges

NORTHEAST

Northeast Foraging: 120 Wild and Flavorful Edibles from Beach Plums to Wineberries by Leda Meredith

Edible Wild Plants: A North American Field Guide to over 200 Natural Foods by Thomas Elias and Peter Dykeman

Incredible Wild Edibles: 36 Plants That Can Change Your Life by Samuel Thayer

SOUTHEAST

Southeast Foraging: 120 Wild and Flavorful Edibles from Angelica to Wild Plums by Chris Bennett

NORTHWEST

Pacific Northwest Foraging: 120 Wild and Flavorful Edibles from Alaska Blueberries to Wild Hazelnuts by Douglas Deur

Foraging the Mountain West: Gourmet Edible Plants, Mushrooms, and Meat by Thomas J. Elpel and Kris Reed

CENTRAL

A Field Guide to Edible Wild Plants: Eastern/Central North America by Lee Allen Peterson and Roger Tory Peterson

Herbalism

The Herbal Medicine-Maker's Handbook: A Home Manual by James Green

A Modern Herbal, Volumes 1 and 2, by Mrs. M. Grieve

The Herbal Handbook: A User's Guide to Medical Herbalism by David Hoffmann

RECISE INDEX

INDEX

Note: Page numbers followed by a "p" refer to photographs. Page numbers followed by a "t" refer to tables.

lamb's-quarter *(Chenopodium album)*
    appearance, 267p
    Boiled Lamb's-Quarter and a
        Dash of Vinegar, 210
    mustard, substitute for, 194
    pickled, 158
    seed collection, 153–54
    See also greens
Laminaria dentigera (kombu), 79, 108, 111
lemon peel/zest, 55, 64, 76, 90
lemony flavors, 74, 78, 79, 103, 122, 127
Lepidium latifolium (perennial pepperweed),
    148, 151, 194
licorice *(Glycyrrhiza glabra),* 89
    See also American licorice
Local Mountains Vinegar Tonic, 258
Lomatium foeniculaceum (desert parsley), 130
London rocket *(Sisymbrium irio),* 157

M

Macrocystis pyrifera (kelp), 79, 108, 110, 111
manzanita berries *(Arctostaphylos manzanita)*
    appearance, 268p
    challenges, 69
    flavor profile, 78, 122, 148
    sugar content, 51
Marrubium vulgare (horehound), 71, 262
mead vinegar, 64–65
    See also alcohol; wine
Mediterranean mustard *(Hirschfeldia incana),*
    153, 157, 182, 200, 251
Melilotus albus (sweet white clover), 78, 90,
    127, 152, 168, 242
Mendocino coast kumbo *(Laminaria
    dentigera),* 79, 108, 111
Mentha aquatica (water mint), 64, 78, 90,
    131, 143, 262
Mexican elder *(Sambucus mexicana),* 94
miner's lettuce *(Claytonia perfoliata)*
    appearance, 268p
    in dressings/pastes, 127, 133
    in salsas, 148, 152
    seeds, 154
Mixed Seasonal Wild Greens and
    Mushrooms Soup, 250

mold
    acidity as deterrent, 50, 88, 229
    appearance, 28
    prevention, 116, 157, 175, 177, 181, 185
    seriousness of, 21, 28, 75
    See also yeast, harmful
morita peppers, 131, 163t, 164, 170, 171
    See also chili peppers
mother of vinegar
    appearance (initial), 14–15
    appearance (optimal), 16, 24,
        27–28p, 31p
    avoiding, 49
    development of, 16, 18, 24
    overview, 14
    storage, 26–28
    variability in, 14
    See also specific vinegars
Mountain Oxymel Aka "Mountain
    Champagne," 261
Mountains Hot Sauce, 168
Mountains Vinegar, 121–22
mugwort *(Artemisia douglasiana)*
    appearance, 268p
    beer vinegar, 27p, 67
    flavoring (optional), 19, 45, 62, 77,
        83, 88
    history of, 10, 74–75
    infusions, 77, 85, 91, 103, 104
    recipes with, 69, 71, 85, 125, 192, 262
    sugar content, 50
    variability in flavor, 11, 121
mushrooms
    adobo, 212p–213
    baby bella (crimini), 206, 250
    dehydrated, 109
    infusions, 79, 109–10p, 152, 164, 210
    jerky, oyster, 232
    lacto-fermented, 226p–227
    Mushrooms and Forest Herbs Salsa, 206
    oyster. *See* oyster mushrooms
    pheasant's back, 187, 227
    preparation tips, 178, 189, 228
    salsa, 206–7p
    shiitake, 226p–227

toxins
    botulism (canning), 33, 179
    herbicides, 1, 97
    on ingredients, 1, 97, 112, 241
    in ingredients, 54–55, 100, 114–16,
        227, 234–35, 250
    tree branches, 100
    See also pasteurization; safety
tree vinegars. *See* pine/fir/spruce vinegars
turkey tail mushrooms *(Trametes versicolor),*
    71–72, 122
Typha latifolia (cattail), 125, 217,
    240p–242

U

Umbellularia californica (California bay leaf),
    77, 78, 79, 230
Unpasteurized Vinegar Starter, 16
Urtica dioica (common stinging nettle), 1, 127,
    133, 157, 158
Using Homemade Vinegar Starter, 30–31p

V

vegetable infusions, 77, 79
    See also infusions
vinaigrettes/dressings (overview), 123–24
vinegar
    acidity. *See* acidity
    active culture, role of, 14
    defined, 13–15
    fermentation. *See* fermentation;
        lacto-fermentation
    flavoring. *See* flavoring
    infusions. *See* infusion recipes; infusions
    main role of, 29, 229
    mother. *See* mother of vinegar
    overview, 29
    spoilage. *See* spoilage
    storage. *See* storage
    vinegar eels, 40
    vinegar flies. *See* fruit flies
Vinegar from Distilled Spirits:
    12-Year-Old Whiskey Vinegar, 48
Vinegar Starter, Unpasteurized, 16
Vinegar to Ingredients Ratio, 79

vinegar, homemade
    accidental, 12–13
    from commercial beers/wines, 42–43
    easiest version, 16–18
    mixing, value of, 30, 73
    overview of, 12–15, 41
    starter, 18, 30–31p, 48, 57–58p
    uniqueness of, 6

W

wakame *(Alaria marginata),* 79, 108, 111
walnuts, 244–47, 246p
wasabi / substitutes for, 135, 147, 158,
    182, 201
    See also chili peppers; hot sauces
Wasabi Ginger Vinegar Sauce, 135
water mint *(Mentha aquatica),* 64, 78, 90,
    131, 143, 262
water, store-bought *vs.* tap, 57, 185
watercress *(Nasturtium officinale),* 269p
whiskey vinegar, 48
white fir *(Abies concolor)*
    appearance, 101p–2p, 105p, 270p
    cold infusion, 81–82, 91, 100–103
    flavor profile, 122
    as garnish, 258
    toxicity concerns, 100
    See also pine/fir/spruce vinegars
white pine *(Pinus strobus),* 100
    See also pine/fir/spruce vinegars
white sage *(Salvia apiana),* 78, 139, 157, 216
white vinegar
    in hot sauce, 161
    for infusions, 76, 91
    mildness of, 29, 163, 190
    recipes with, 83, 85, 135, 214, 243
    for starter, 48
    as substitute ingredient, 128, 129, 147,
        148, 171, 209
    substitutions for, 91
white/yellow mustard *(Sinapis alba),*
    129, 158
wild barley *(Hordeum spontaneum),* 112, 214
wild carrot *(Daucus carota),* 98, 132, 175,
    182, 204

ABOUT THE AUTHOR

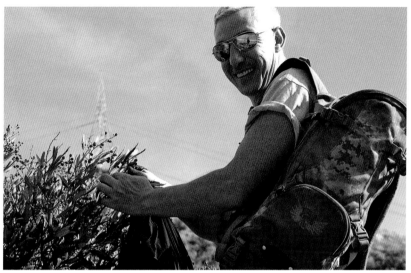

Pascal Baudar is the author of three previous books: *Wildcrafted Fermentation* (2020), *The Wildcrafting Brewer* (2018), and *The New Wildcrafted Cuisine* (2016). A self-described "culinary alchemist," he leads classes in traditional food preservation techniques. Through his business, Urban Outdoor Skills, he has introduced thousands of home cooks, celebrity chefs, and foodies to the flavors offered by their wild landscapes. In 2014, Baudar was named one of the most influential local tastemakers by *Los Angeles Magazine*.

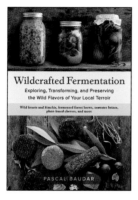
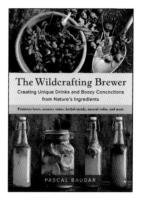
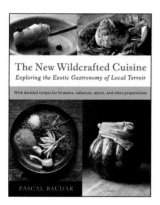
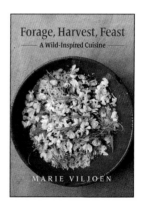
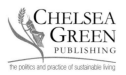

the politics and practice of sustainable living

CHELSEA GREEN PUBLISHING

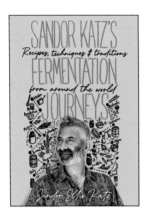

SANDOR KATZ'S FERMENTATION JOURNEYS
Recipes, Techniques, and Traditions
from around the World
SANDOR ELLIX KATZ
9781645020349
Hardcover

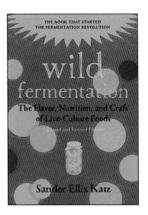

WILD FERMENTATION
The Flavor, Nutrition, and Craft
of Live-Culture Foods,
Updated and Revised Edition
SANDOR ELLIX KATZ
9781603586283
Paperback

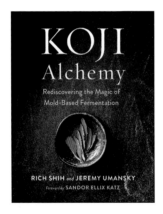

KOJI ALCHEMY
Rediscovering the Magic of
Mold-Based Fermentation
RICH SHIH and JEREMY UMANSKY
9781603588683
Hardcover

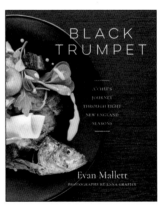

BLACK TRUMPET
A Chef's Journey Through
Eight New England Seasons
EVAN MALLETT
9781603586504
Hardcover

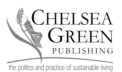

CHELSEA
GREEN
PUBLISHING

the politics and practice of sustainable living

For more information,
visit **www.chelseagreen.com**.